The Doctor Is In

THE DOCTOR IS IN

The compelling (and true) story of a McMaster Medical School graduate

By Dr. Bobbi Lancaster

Foreword by Dr. Paul O'Byrne

The Doctor Is In

This work is a memoir. The stories have been retrieved from the author's memory of the events. In some cases, names have been changed or abbreviated in an effort to respect privacy. However, most of the individuals are readily identifiable because of their close relationship to the author. Every effort was made to portray them in an honest and positive manner. First do no harm—borrowed from the Hippocratic Oath—was the rule adhered to when writing about others.

All rights reserved

Copyright © 2020 Bobbi Lancaster

ISBN: 978-1-7334635-3-9

No part of this publication may be reproduced, stored in a retrieval system, or transmitted in any form or by any means electronic, mechanical, photocopying, recording, or otherwise, without the written permission of the author or publisher.

The Doctor Is In

By the Same Author

The Red Light Runner

Putting Down Roots

My Friend Flutter

From Paris I Came

Backyard Adventures

The Doctor Is In

Dedication

I am forever grateful for all my amazing teachers.

The Doctor Is In

TABLE OF CONTENTS

Foreword..ix

Preface...xv

One: A Shaky Start....................................1

Two: Doctoring Is Not For Me.....................9

Three: May I Quit Now?............................17

Four: Inside The Ropes............................23

Five: My Freshman Year...........................45

Six: Early Experiences..............................53

Seven: Clerkship—Care For A Smoke?.......57

Eight: No Thanks, Dr. Freud.....................67

Nine: Not Ready For Prime Time...............73

Ten: Lost But Not Forgotten......................81

Eleven: A Second Chance.........................87

Twelve: Clerkship Again—Raising Lazarus.....93

Thirteen: Zebras I Have Come To Know..........113

Fourteen: Dr. Paul O'Byrne And Me............127

Fifteen: Breaking Up Is Hard To Do............141

Sixteen: Pursuing Excellence—One Patient At A Time..................169

Seventeen: Stormy Days..................189

Eighteen: Greener Pastures..................197

Nineteen: Gone Too Soon..................205

Twenty: The Heart Of The Matter..................211

Twenty-One: Advocacy..................217

Twenty-Two: Flying Too Close To The Sun....227

Twenty-Three: Finding Peace..................237

Twenty-Four: Time To Say Good-Bye..................239

About The Author..................249

Acknowledgements..................253

The Doctor Is In

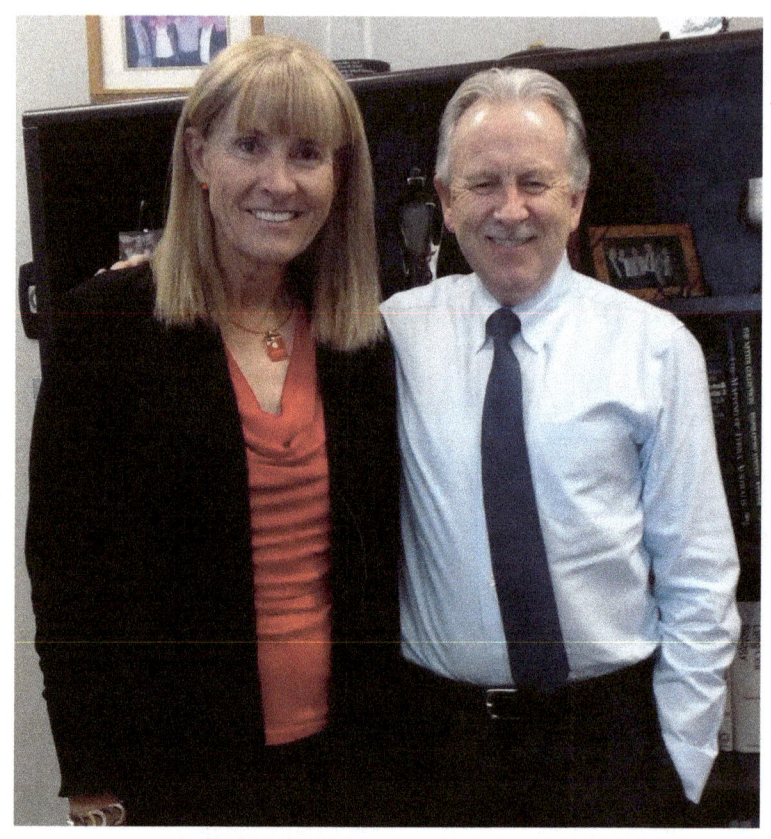

The Doctor Is In

FOREWORD BY DR. PAUL O'BYRNE

In September of 1969, the first class of medical students was welcomed to McMaster University in Hamilton, Ontario. It was here that the founding dean, Dr. John Evans, and four colleagues—Drs. Anderson, Mustard, Spaulding and Walsh—reshaped the entire model of medical education. They became known as the Founding Fathers. At the time, their work was considered risky and controversial. They recruited science and non-science students from diverse educational backgrounds; had them work in small groups; trusted they would find and evaluate the evidence needed to make sound clinical judgments, and engaged them early with patients. There were no lectures or formal examinations. To top it all off, the school was the first to offer a three-year curriculum instead of the standard four years, which had been the norm in medical schools in Canada and the rest of the world.

In 1971, Robert (Bob) Lancaster applied to McMaster Medical School. I suspect this was not because of its revolutionary pedagogy. Rather, he had an undergraduate degree in biology, and his family lived in Hamilton. Bob was accepted into the fourth medical class and graduated, not in the expected three years but in 1978, after six long years. The reasons for this delay are detailed in this book, a remarkable story of challenge and resilience. Robert is now Dr. Bobbi Lancaster—a transgender woman—and one of the most outstanding medical graduates that McMaster has ever produced. However, I'm getting ahead of myself.

I had arrived at McMaster University in July 1977—initially to train in Internal Medicine—after completing my medical degree and a couple of years of postgraduate training in Dublin, Ireland. Robert and I initially met in the fall of 1978, when he was doing a mandatory medicine rotation as part of his Family Medicine residency. This meeting occurred in a somewhat unusual clinical setting. The medical school and its hospital partner had recently decided to develop a ward for the acute care of medical patients—and put it under the control of the Department of Family Medicine! As the chief resident, I was assigned to supervise three first-year Family Medicine interns during their rotation on this experimental ward. It was a thirty-bed unit with a high level of clinical acuity. In this type of environment you got to know, very quickly, the acumen of the newly minted physicians under your command, as well as your own abilities and limitations. Bob turned out to be a superb young doctor who faced and triumphed over a series of obstacles that would have overwhelmed most of us.

The Doctor Is In describes Bob's early years as a McMaster medical student. As with most other learners, their first exposure to patients usually invokes the strongest memories, and this was particularly true for him. These memories include seeing a patient die on the operating table during a first opportunity to scrub and assist a surgeon, as well as experiencing the elation of delivering a baby. The challenges all medical students face are told honestly, including the decision that Bob made to drop out of medical school.

This book also eloquently illustrates the vital importance of good mentorship at critical stages in a young person's life. The support and timely advice that Bob received from his assigned student advisor—Dr.Ron McAuley—was life-altering. A family physician and an educator at the medical school, Dr. Ron helped guide Robert through the chaos of leaving and ultimately re-entering the program. This chapter of the book forcefully communicates, especially for me, the need to focus on medical student wellness during this immensely challenging time of learning—something that most medical schools have not, until recently, taken much note of. I believe this is changing and not a moment too soon.

The Doctor Is In is also a vivid and compelling telling of the life of a young family physician. It describes both the joys and the stresses of trying to manage a hectic clinical practice while at the same time attempting to balance life as a husband and father of young children.

Unfortunately, the families of most physicians pay a high price during clinical training and while a practice is being developed.

During our time together on the ward, I learned that Bob was not only a skilled young physician but also a superb competitive golfer. He had won many tournaments and club championships, and had captained the McMaster varsity golf team to two OUAA victories. Bob was very modest about these achievements and had never discussed them during our interactions together on the wards. This athletic ability played an important role later on in this extraordinary life story—when Bob transitioned to life as Bobbi.

I lost track of Bob after he left Hamilton to move to Arizona. So it was a wonderful surprise when a member of the Dean's advancement team, Ann Brodie, mentioned that she'd had a chance to meet Dr. Bobbi—an interesting McMaster Medical School alumna—over lunch in Arizona in the spring of 2017. At that time, I had rather recently been appointed Dean. Ann suggested that I meet with Bobbi the next time she visited Hamilton. Ann also mentioned that Bobbi was a transgender woman and I would remember her as Robert Lancaster from the 1970s. Now my curiosity was really piqued and added to my desire to meet Bobbi and learn about her life story.

We met in my office (the picture of that meeting is included in the book), and it was as though the intervening almost four decades had disappeared. Bobbi was just as charming, engaging and joyful to meet with—just like the Bob I remembered from years ago. And the story of her transition, as well as the remarkable events surrounding her career as a professional women's golfer—competing against some of the very best young players in the world—was spell-binding.

During our one-hour meeting, it occurred to me that having Bobbi speak to our second-year medical students at our annual "Founders Dinner" might inspire all in attendance. I asked if she would consider returning to Hamilton to provide the keynote address and Bobbi readily agreed.

The event was a stunning success. I have attended many of these medical student dinners over my years at McMaster University, and I have never seen such a positive reaction to a speaker as occurred that evening. Bobbi's life is quite unique, as you will see in this book. That night, she told her story in a way that was highly engaging, often amusing, and full of insight. The students were entranced and gave Bobbi a prolonged standing ovation at the end of the presentation—one richly deserved! My wife, Irene, who attended the dinner, said later that it was the best talk she had ever heard from a physician (including me!).

The Doctor Is In is an engaging and entertaining read. Beautifully written and full of practical life lessons, this book explores: the challenges of medical school; the essence of being a doctor; the need to try to satisfy competing family responsibilities; the reality of being transgender, and the emotional trauma that results from navigating these experiences.

In summary, the story of Bobbi—a proud and resilient graduate of McMaster Medical School—is one of hope, courage, determination and optimism. This book reinforces my own view that in spite of the many difficulties faced while completing training to become a physician, the joys experienced in this profession make it all worthwhile.

PREFACE

I have a confession to make. In the fall of 1971, when I applied for admission to McMaster Medical School, I knew almost nothing about the curriculum. Of course I'd heard the school was a little different, and you could earn your degree in three years. But it was my first choice because I was familiar with McMaster University, and was enrolled in its honors biology program. The campus was in my home town of Hamilton, and I could continue to live with my parents—avoiding the expense of a dormitory room.

The medical school was different alright, but I never considered it special at the time. I was too busy being stressed out of my mind as I tried to navigate the self-directed nightmare. Mostly, I felt like a didactically-trained square trying to fit into a Socratic hole.

In spite of a personal meltdown and leave of absence, I eventually graduated and thought I would never look back. Many years passed. I relocated to Arizona, and couldn't help but notice that my alma mater was rising in the world rankings. This unusual learning model was now being considered one of the greatest breakthroughs in education in the past hundred years. It was being copied by other medical schools around the globe, and the original visionaries were now revered and called the Founding Fathers.

I caught myself bragging that I was a graduate of McMaster—the internationally renowned medical school near Toronto (no one in Phoenix seemed to know where Hamilton is located). "I've been trained at an iconic school," I'd declare, in an effort to bolster my bona fides. However, I still shuddered when I thought about the actual experience.

Three years ago, after a series of unbelievable twists and turns, Dr. Paul O'Byrne—the current dean of the school—rediscovered me in Arizona. He had been the chief resident during my internal medicine rotation in 1978. When you dive into this book, you will learn he made an offer I couldn't refuse. He requested I deliver a keynote address to the current students, faculty and staff.

In preparing my speech, I had to face my lingering antipathy toward the program. I also embarked on a fact-finding mission, searching for comments from other graduates. I was surprised to discover there were no other relevant books, papers or publications. Nothing!

It was at that moment I decided to write about my experiences as a student. The history is simply too important to be left undocumented. *The Doctor Is In* is my attempt to memorialize the early days, and demonstrate the profound impact this training has had on my personal growth and development—even to this day.

After a great deal of thought, I have concluded that my early difficulties were not the fault of the program. They were the result of my immaturity and the myriad personal problems I was grappling with at the time.

While writing the first draft of this book, I felt intense moments of sadness when I stared at their names on my computer screen: Drs. Kemp, Evans, Spaulding, Mustard, Walsh, Anderson, McAuley, Rudnick, Barrows, Sackett, and Shirley Hurst—nurse practitioner extraordinaire. And there are too many more to mention!

I knew them all. They were my teachers and mentors, and they are all gone. I would have liked to interview them and properly thank them for all they did for me… and perhaps for you as well. But they have passed on—every last one of them. I had postponed this project a little too long.

I'm grateful and proud to be a McMaster Medical School graduate.

And now I invite you to enjoy my stories.

The Doctor Is In

The Doctor Is In

CHAPTER ONE
A SHAKY START

It was as sudden as it was unexpected—a violent unleashing of blood—striking the overhead operating room light, like an angry slap. The brief eruption appeared to end before it started. But not before the surgeon's face and scrubs were splattered, marking him as the perpetrator. The scene looked surreal—straight out of a Jackson Pollock painting. There was a collective gasp, a moment of silence and then organized chaos.

I had been there to observe my first surgery as a newbie medical student. Now I was at the center of the incident: a retractor in one hand holding open the surgical site; a suction device in the other as I unsuccessfully tried to reduce the now sizeable puddle of blood in the abdomen. The family doctor, who was serving as first assistant, was suctioning too and blotting frantically in the hope of providing a glimpse of the epicenter.

Only minutes before, the surgeon had been describing his approach as he cut through various layers of tissue. His mission was to locate an enormous abdominal aortic aneurysm and bypass it with a graft. He was asking me to name the structures encountered along the way. I could not identify even one landmark, which was understandable: I was a freshman just starting my third week at McMaster Medical School. The program involved its students in real-life medical situations right from the get-go, and I was proud that I had at least mastered the pre-operative ritual of scrubbing, gown and gloving.

This did not stop the surgeon from reprimanding me about my lack of preparation. He told me I had better visit the cadaver lab and read *Gray's Anatomy* before I ever enter his operating theater again.

I felt myself withdrawing—I never did take criticism very well. I couldn't help but notice the surgeon's gloved hands. There was a not-so-subtle tremor, and I wondered if anyone else had noticed. Still stinging from his scolding, I glanced over the barrier in the direction of the anesthesiologist. He was busily injecting some medication into an IV port. The patient—a jolly, red-faced man—was intubated, and his face was turned toward me.

I had enjoyed meeting Mr. Armstrong yesterday afternoon, during which time he'd introduced me to his wife and told me about his life as a steel worker. It was an opportunity to practice my history-taking and physical examination skills. My nervousness was obvious, but his jocular nature put me at ease.

In the early 1970s, it was customary to admit patients to the hospital the day before elective surgery. Routine labs, a chest X-ray, and an EKG were ordered to be certain there were no unexpected issues that might impact surgery. I discovered that this retired laborer was being treated for high blood pressure. He was also a drinker, a pack-a-day smoker, and possessed a very ample, hard-earned beer belly.

The aneurysm had been found by his family doctor. He had been teaching another medical student how to perform a thorough abdominal exam when they heard a swooshing noise—a bruit—made by the turbulent flow of blood as it jetted through an enlarged aorta. It was an unmistakable and quite alarming sound.

And now everything had converged to this moment in time—a true life-or-death emergency. The room felt like it was spinning. Urgent commands filled the claustrophobic space: lower the head of the table; order blood; establish a third intravenous; run in some Ringers—full bore; call for another surgeon; notify the intensive care; speak with the family. I was frozen in place as I watched beads of perspiration collect on the old surgeon's forehead. His glasses fogged as he clutched instruments in his now wildly tremulous hands, blindly trying to find the proximal end of the aorta. Alarm bells were sounding from all directions.

I remember glancing at Mr. Armstrong again. He was still facing me—white as a ghost—and appeared quite peaceful in his anesthetized state.

Nothing I had ever experienced had prepared me for this moment.

Of course the patient coded—a cardiac arrest. While the newly arrived Arrest Team performed CPR and defibrillation, the work below continued. There was a much better view of the ruptured aneurysm because almost all the patient's blood now resided in soaked sponges, towels, suction bottles, uniforms, the overhead lamp and even the floor. The situation reminded me of a crude joke—handed down by tough-as-nails surgeons to generations of medical students before me: "Don't panic when you encounter dramatic bleeding...because all bleeding stops eventually." Except this was not a joking matter.

Mr. Armstrong mattered, and his wife and family were waiting for news.

The tattered remnants of the aorta were replaced by a graft, but the patient remained in cardiac arrest. He was moved to the ICU because, "no one dies in the operating room." Every conceivable resuscitative maneuver was employed as the well-rehearsed team members followed their preplanned decision tree. I observed the entire endurance event.

After an hour, initial heroic efforts gave way to exhaustion. Mr. Armstrong's pupils were fixed and dilated—it had become an exercise in futility. The code was called, and the patient was pronounced dead. The team dispersed as quickly as they had appeared, so they could attend to other patients. They'd conducted themselves in a professional, business-like manner.

The family doctor and I retreated to the surgeon's lounge and quickly changed into fresh scrubs. Mrs. Armstrong and the other family members had been directed to a private room and were anxiously awaiting a report. I asked if I could tag along.

The gray-haired surgeon was in the change room too—alone with his thoughts—still wearing his soiled uniform. He appeared small and defeated. I touched his shoulder and said I was sorry. He did not look up and remained frozen in place. I later heard that he retired the next day. After too many years of extraordinary service, this was his last case.

A social worker, the head nurse and a pastoral staff member escorted us to the door. The family doctor knocked and we entered—an entourage—and were greeted with teary-eyed but hopeful expressions. He explained, using medical terms, that there had been complications and uncontrollable bleeding. Their loved one—

a husband, father, papa, and friend to many—was dead. The doctor expressed his sadness and awkwardly looked at the floor.

There was a collective gasp quickly followed by a shriek, and then the floodgates opened. The family gathered around Mrs. Armstrong and held her tight. The doctor motioned to me that we should leave.

I had been a fly on the wall, holding back my emotions and forbidding myself to cry. However, I could not stop the tears from running down my face. Mrs. Armstrong noticed my movement toward the door and broke free from her family's embrace. We hugged for the longest time. It was as much for her as it was for me.

And then it was over. We left the family in the capable hands of the grief counselors. While walking back to the change room, the doctor asked if I was alright and then admonished me. "You will need to learn to keep your emotions in check," he lectured, "or you will be an ineffective physician." I nodded. However, I wasn't certain I agreed with his advice.

After showering—in an attempt to cleanse myself from this traumatic day—I emerged from the hospital. A beautiful sunset unfolded in front of my eyes. However, it was impossible to enjoy. I felt sick to my stomach, and there was a busy day planned for tomorrow.

What had I gotten myself in to?

Did I really have what it would take to be a physician?

Yet, how could I quit the program after just a few weeks and face my parents? What would I say to my fiancée, Mary Jo, and her family? Their collective disappointment would be more than I could handle.

On the other hand, I wasn't sure that I could emotionally survive another event like this one. I'd never seen a person die before.

As I slowly drove home, my thoughts wandered back to another time and place. I was trying to make sense of this career decision, especially given my dislike of doctors and everything about them when I was young.

How had I arrived at this place?

The Doctor Is In

CHAPTER TWO
DOCTORING IS NOT FOR ME

The exam room door flew open with a bang, and I ran to the crowded reception area. My mother followed quickly in an effort to catch up. In my moment of anger, I stopped abruptly and yelled out for all to hear. "That man put his finger up my butt and hurt me a lot! I'm never coming back to this doctor again!"

Everyone was startled to attention, while Mom flushed with embarrassment. I was only six, but I could run like the wind. After loudly voicing my indignation one more time, I raced out the office door while looking over my shoulder—to see if Mother was in pursuit.

And I ran smack into a huge metal pole that supported the only stoplight in this tiny main-street town. Witnesses said that I dropped like a stone as blood bubbled from a rapidly growing lump on my forehead. Bystanders carried me back to the same examination room I had just exited. Then the doctor proceeded to hurt me all over again—pouring stinging liquid repeatedly on my wound. I screamed at the top of my lungs.

Eventually, the sobbing ended and my breathing calmed down. Mom held my hand as I lay on the table. I became aware of the smells all around me.

I'm not certain what chemicals created the odor, but they stamped a permanent olfactory memory on my young, impressionable brain. Many years later, I occasionally catch a whiff of an antiseptic and am instantly transported back to the doctor's office of my childhood.

The visit to Dr. Betts had been necessary because, for months, I'd been having extremely painful bowel movements with bleeding, and Mom was concerned. The doctor explained I had an anal fissure, a tear, likely caused by a large, hard bowel movement months before. He prescribed softeners and laxatives to aid in the healing process. Why this gruff former army doctor, with his overly large hands, had to stick a finger up my rear made no sense. He had already told us what was wrong. His unnecessary examination simply tore me again.

This was my first memory of going to a doctor. Up until then, Mom—with the help of old family remedies—had treated all my ailments: red measles, German measles, mumps, chicken pox, poison ivy, and a cut on my leg. She used Vicks and steam for my asthma, mustard or onion poultices depending on the condition, warm compresses for boils, and Mercurochrome for abrasions. Mom even fixed my right arm after it got caught in the revolving rollers of the ringer washing machine during a moment of play.

Every week I received cod liver oil, vitamins, and milk of magnesia to keep me well. These preventive measures were clearly not working because I contracted most of the childhood illnesses common at the time. Thankfully, I did not acquire polio, an illness that was still not eradicated in the early 1950s. My father had been stricken with it in high school and luckily had made a full recovery.

Dr. Betts and I were not finished with each other yet. Our dramatic and final meeting occurred a year later when he performed a tonsillectomy on me and my younger brother, Ron—on the same day. My memory of the event is somewhat vague for reasons that will become obvious. To this day, I think the operations were done at our home on the kitchen table. However, my now ninety-year-old mom thinks they might have been done at Dr. Betts' office, but her memory is understandably becoming a little fuzzy too.

Ron went first as I nervously awaited my turn. At the conclusion of the brief procedure, he looked alright; nothing ever seemed to bother him. However, my heart was pounding, and I did not have the appearance of a brave older brother. I remember my terror as Dr. Betts placed an ether-soaked cloth—with its unforgettable odor—over my face. I gripped the edge of the table for dear life.

The Doctor Is In

When I awoke, the first person I spied was Ron. He was enjoying his reward—a bowl of vanilla ice cream. On the other hand, I was struggling with intense throat pain and repeatedly had to swallow some nasty tasting saliva. My distress continued throughout the night and all the next day. Overwhelming weakness was followed by nausea and then explosive vomiting. Everything in the room became covered with my blood. A suture that should have tied-off my tonsillar artery had come undone, and I was bleeding to death.

Panic ensued: an hysterical phone call to the doctor; the request for a police escort; drifting in and out of consciousness to the sound of a siren; an ambulance racing through the rural countryside to Chatham, and arriving an hour later at St. Joseph's Hospital. Just in the nick of time, I was rushed to the operating room. After multiple transfusions and a procedure, the bleeding was staunched and my life was saved.

The next day I enjoyed a bowl of vanilla ice cream too.

My relationship with Dr. Betts was over, but there was still Dr. Rivers to contend with. He was the dentist, or so he claimed, and I had lots of cavities to keep him busy. Every time my mom took me to his office, he found two or three more.

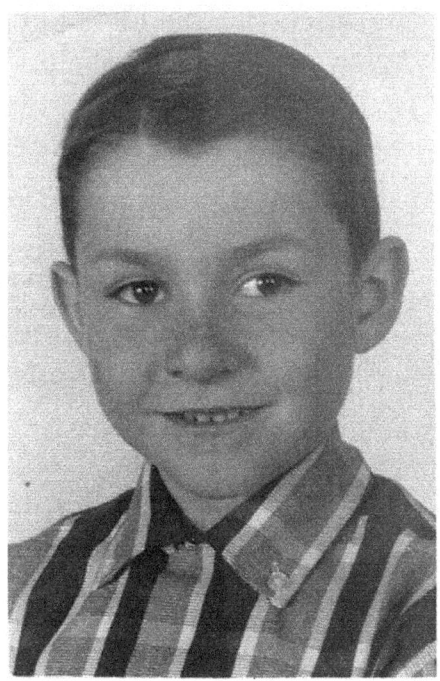

Bob Lancaster (eight years old)

Dr. Rivers tilted me back in a chair. I don't recall receiving any local anesthetic, and he never explained what he was doing. He spun the drill by rocking his foot back and forth on a floor-mounted metal plate, like the old Singer sewing machine my mom owned. At the start of each procedure, Dr. Rivers was full of energy. The drill spun quickly, and there was almost no pain. However, as his leg fatigued, the drill slowed and the discomfort was unbearable. He seemed oblivious to my squirming. Even to this day when I visit my modern dentist for routine cleaning, I am a nervous, fidgeting mess.

Except for the doctors, this idyllic little town—Ridgetown—was a magical place. I became engaged in many happy activities: collecting and studying butterflies; excelling at multiple sports; becoming a skilled pianist; delivering newspapers; serving as an altar boy at St. Michael's Catholic Church. I was an above-average student, but my writing was illegible. The nuns administered frequent scolding and remedial homework to improve my penmanship.

When I was ten, in spite of my protestations, we moved from Ridgetown to the big city of Hamilton two hours away. There were five of us now: Mom, Dad, me, Ron and my four-year-old sister, Sandy. My father had found a better paying job as a tax auditor. We were told there would be great schools, improved healthcare, and more career opportunities. I was skeptical.

However, many good things did happen in short order: my new brother, Ken, was born in 1961; work as a caddy replaced my old newspaper delivery job; my piano studies with the Royal Conservatory of Music continued; school was easy; Regina Mundi Church welcomed my altar-boy skills, and I became a champion junior golfer.

However, my asthma and seasonal allergies had become problematic. It was time to meet our new family physician, Dr. Murphy. His office smelled just like Dr. Betts'. Dr. Murphy was younger and had one large eyebrow that occupied his entire forehead. And he was the original sourpuss. No matter how nice the weather or how well the local sports team performed, Dr. Murphy had something negative to say.

He treated my asthma by prescribing an inhaler and allergy shots. These weekly painful injections went on for years, and I amused myself by playing a private game: I was determined to get Dr. Murphy to smile. In spite of my best efforts, I'm sad to say that the shots were ineffective, and his downturned mouth never did change expression.

At this point, I had come to the following conclusions about doctors and dentists: they were all gruff and uncaring; inflicted pain in a detached fashion; did not appear to enjoy their work; were always rushed, and their offices all had the same unappealing, antiseptic smell.

Even though I was in my early teens, I was thinking about what I might be when I grew up: a priest, a concert pianist, a professional golfer, or maybe a butterfly expert. Yes, I would be a renowned lepidopterist and spend my life doing field work and teaching.

One thing was certain though. I was never going to be a doctor. I could not imagine joining the likes of Drs. Betts, Rivers, and Murphy.

The Doctor Is In

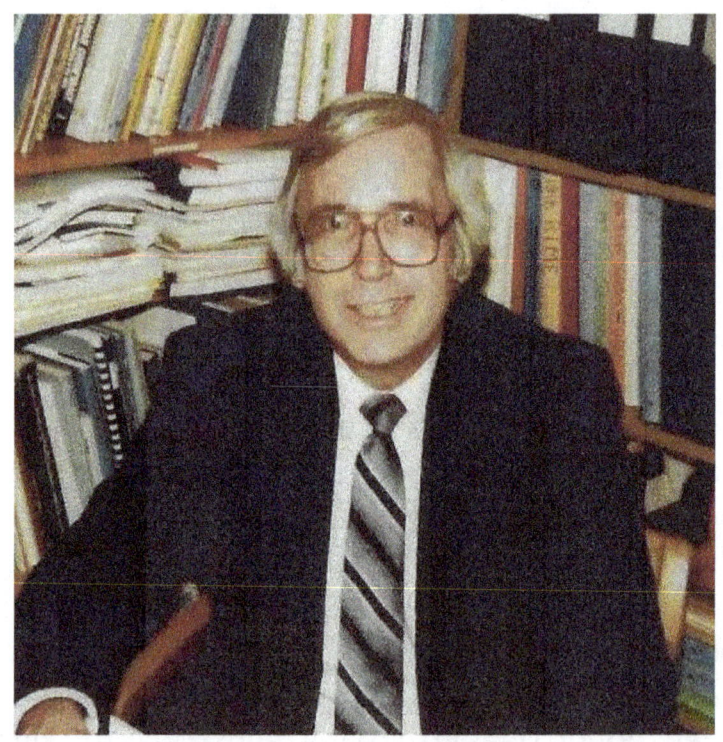

Dr. Ron McAuley

CHAPTER THREE
MAY I QUIT NOW?

Dr. Ron McAuley listened attentively as I related the events surrounding the death of the patient during surgery. In dramatic fashion, I described the elderly surgeon's tremulous hands and the pandemonium that was unleashed when the aneurysm was accidently nicked. The memory of the discussion with the family still brought tears to my eyes. I wanted to quit.

Every medical student was assigned a mentor, and it was my good fortune to have been placed with Dr. McAuley. He was a seasoned family physician and an extraordinary teacher. His kindness was unmatched. I had not anticipated meeting with him so early in the program. In fact I didn't really understand the point of a mentor or counselor, given the fact I considered myself self-reliant and had always tried to solve my own problems.

He changed the topic and asked me about my family. I told him that I had been born in 1950, the oldest of four children, and was the first Lancaster to attend university in anyone's memory. He learned there was tension in our home because my father was a violent alcoholic who frequently beat my mother and brother. I recounted how I'd recently physically confronted my father—

threatened to kill him—because he had assaulted Mom one time too many. My dad promised he would never drink again and would lead a life I would be proud of—he said he didn't want to lose me. We were in the watch-and-wait phase of the mess at the moment.

Dr. McAuley had a way of asking questions. It was like he had administered a truth serum of some sort, and I just kept blabbering on. Dr. Ron, as he liked to be called, asked what I liked to do when I wasn't studying. I told him about my infatuation with nature; the treasured microscope I had received for Christmas; my study of butterflies since I was eight; the multi-sport athletic awards; my golfing prowess and many victories; the love I had for the piano, and all the various summer jobs I'd worked since I was seven.

Most of all, I told Dr. McAuley how much I liked helping people. It started when I was very young. I had noticed the old couple next door having trouble raking their leaves—they appeared unsteady and stumbled several times. I took the rake in my six-year-old hands and cleaned their yard. They were so surprised and appreciative! Of course I cleared the snow from their sidewalk too until we moved away. They told my parents all about my kindness and offered money, which I refused. This was the first solid bit of evidence that I would be a lousy businessman.

The Doctor Is In

My story was interrupted when Dr. McAuley held up his hand, cleared his throat, and leaned toward me. He told me that he was really sorry I had been part of such an unusual and horrible surgical misadventure, one that would probably never happen again for the rest of my professional career.

He followed by insisting that, in his opinion, I would be an incredible doctor someday, and he urged me not to quit.

I appreciated his comments. However, I still had doubts about my suitability and told him the following story. Several months earlier, I had worked in the pro shop at Chedoke Civic Golf Course. It was my summer job, and everyone knew I was starting medical school in September. In fact, the regulars were already calling me "Doc."

One particularly hot afternoon, I had just finished my shift when I noticed a commotion on the tenth tee. I walked down from the shop to find a circle of people—three or four deep—surrounding a fallen golfer. It was the elderly Mr. Turnbull, and he was unconscious. Everyone was standing and gawking, including me, while his daughter was yelling and pleading for help. She was pushing on his chest and blowing into her father's mouth.

There were no cell phones in the early seventies, and so someone ran to the shop to call for an ambulance. I did not know CPR and had no clue about what to do. I told myself that I should have burst through the onlookers and asked the daughter how I could help. I could have done something. However, for some reason, I held back. I hoped no one would recognize me and push me into the spotlight. I felt ashamed.

The paramedics finally arrived—after too long a time—and transported the lifeless body to the hospital. I later learned that Mr. Turnbull had died from a coronary thrombosis... whatever that was.

I offered this story to Dr. McAuley as further evidence that I did not have the courage or the character required to be a doctor. There was a note of exasperation in his voice, and he reprimanded me for being too hard on myself. He suggested we meet again in a month and urged me to engage in more positive self-talk.

That was the end of our first of many meetings. I would continue to study hard, self-criticize less and avail myself of every learning experience that presented itself. However, there was one thing I promised myself. Dr. Ron McAuley—this soul whisperer—would never discover my most guarded secret. I was a transgender individual. I cross-dressed. When I was fourteen, a priest

I'd confided in told me my behavior was sinful. He prescribed a lengthy penance that I felt was unjustified. I was being punished for the sin of being me.

The pastor's condemnation of my behavior had weighed heavily on me. I made every effort to stop cross-dressing, and failed over and over. I became convinced I was going to hell.

So, I tried to be a normal male and hid my truth from everyone, including Mary Jo. Our wedding day in December of 1972 was rapidly approaching. I continued to perform many generous and kind acts on a daily basis, in the hope that God was watching and would give me a reprieve.

I'd never heard of a transgender physician. I feared that this perceived personal flaw alone was probably disqualifying.

The Doctor Is In

CHAPTER FOUR
INSIDE THE ROPES

"Have you ever wanted to attend medical school, even for just one day? Well, today you are in luck, because I'm inviting you to follow me around. Remember that my school—McMaster—is no ordinary place of learning. Its curriculum is a radical departure from all the usual traditions. I'll explain shortly.

"I've only completed my first few weeks of study and you can relax, because I won't be observing a surgery today. Given the disaster that occurred during the first and only procedure I'd ever observed, I have no intention of stepping foot in an operating room again—until it becomes mandatory later in my training.

"Today I have a tutorial group meeting, a planned visit to the anatomy lab, and then I'll spend the afternoon at Dr. Bob Kemp's office. He's a family physician whose practice is in the nearby town of Stoney Creek. I visit there once a week—all part of my real world clinical training. This early exposure to patients, right from the beginning, is unique to McMaster.

"Before we get started, let's grab a cup of coffee as we drive from downtown Hamilton toward the university. Let me fill you in on some history.

"McMaster was established in 1887—a Baptist-sponsored undergraduate institution—and it focused on theology and the arts. Initially located in Toronto, where the school outgrew its footprint, McMaster was moved to Hamilton in 1930. Here it became a public place of learning and quickly gained prominence in the fields of science, engineering, social science, and later business.

"By the 1960s, Hamilton was one of the major manufacturing hubs in Canada—a steel town—and many of its citizens were immigrants from Europe. Proud of their origins, they were equally appreciative to live and raise their families in this bustling lunch-bucket town.

"Dr. Henry Thode, the President of the University during that time, hatched a bold plan that would put McMaster on the international academic map. He envisioned a medical school. However, there was heavy lifting to do: securing funding; finding a space to situate the medical center; obtaining zoning changes and permits; choosing an architect, and hiring a dean—just to name a few.

"We're on Sterling Avenue now and McMaster University Medical Center—MUMC to everyone connected—is just ahead and to the left. I'm going to pull over to the curb and stop. I want you to look at this neighborhood—Westdale—

and appreciate the mature trees, manicured lawns, classic architecture and obvious pride of ownership. And let's pretend that you can see the McMaster Sunken Gardens just over there: a place of unsurpassed beauty, the location for many weddings, and a point of civic pride for all Hamiltonians. Now imagine Dr. Thode and his team requesting expropriation of ninety homes in this toney neighborhood, and the bulldozing of the Garden—all for the purpose of building a medical school. It was like a bomb had gone off in the community.

"To make matters worse, Dr. Thode produced an artist's rendition and a model of what the new school would look like. A famous architect—Ed Zeidler—had designed an incredibly functional and adaptive building. However, it was a monstrosity—an example of a style popular at the time called brutalism. The locals revolted.

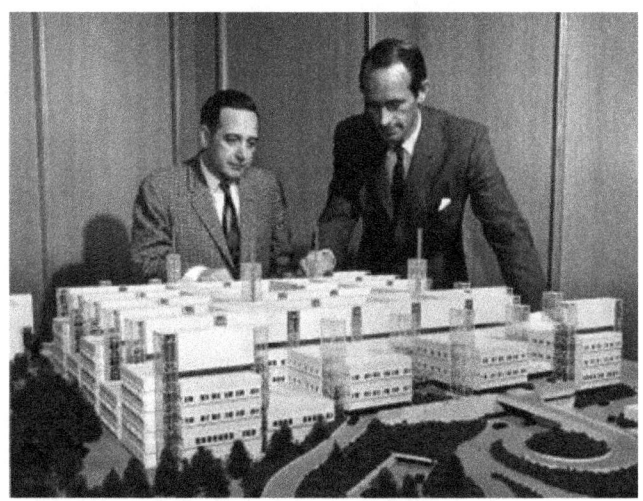

Ed Zeidler (left) with Dr. Evans

"It didn't help either that Dr. Thode made an unusual choice for his first dean—Dr. John Evans.

"He was barely thirty-five years old, a Rhode's Scholar, and he had some wild ideas about educating medical students: they would not be required to have a science background; more than their GPA would be used as an admission requirement; the usual four-year program would be shortened to three, with the elimination of summer breaks; there would be no lectures or exams, and the students would essentially design their own curriculum. Tutorial group meetings, utilizing a problem-based learning model, were proposed as the core of the program.

"Dr. Evans had already trotted out these musings

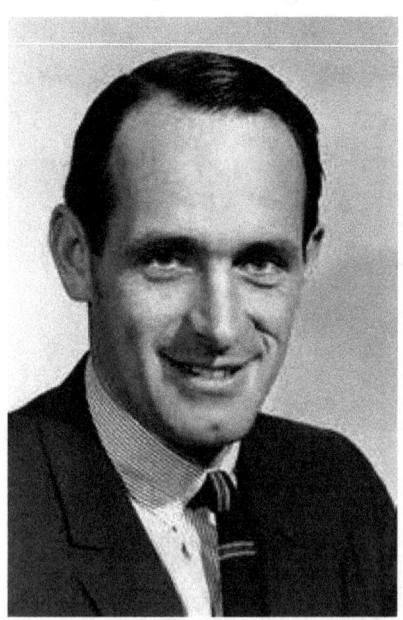

Dr. John Evans

to his alma mater—the University of Toronto—when he applied to be their new dean. He and his radical ideas were rejected.

"As you might expect, there were many divisive community meetings and enormous pushback. However, it was Dr. Bill Walsh—a beloved Westdale internist—who saved the day. He had been the senior resident during Dr. Evans' medical rotation in Toronto, and his people skills had made a lasting impresssion.

"This charismatic leader was well respected. Bill was a resident of the neighborhood, a good listener, and a consensus builder. People would gravitate to him because he always found a way for everyone to win.

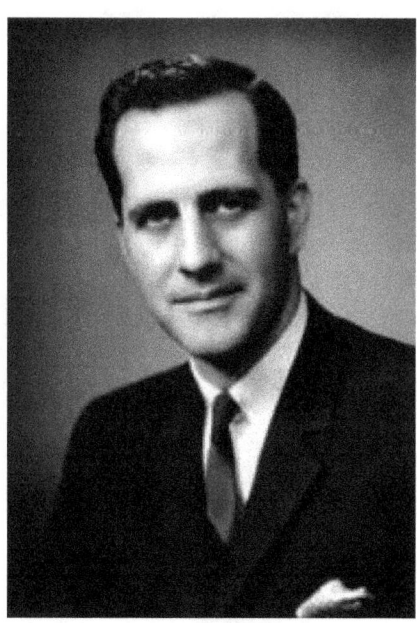

Dr. Bill Walsh

"Without Dr. Walsh's influence, I don't think the dream would have gotten off the ground.

"Once it became clear that the school would be built, Dr. Evans assembled a core of other like-minded individuals he had met during his University of Toronto training.

"There was Dr. Fraser Mustard—an internationally acclaimed blood clot researcher and an imposing figure—who could transform a student into a jellyfish with one glance. He was an outspoken critic of contemporary medical education and its lack of a holistic approach. He felt that the social issues contributing to disease were being completely ignored. Dr. Mustard

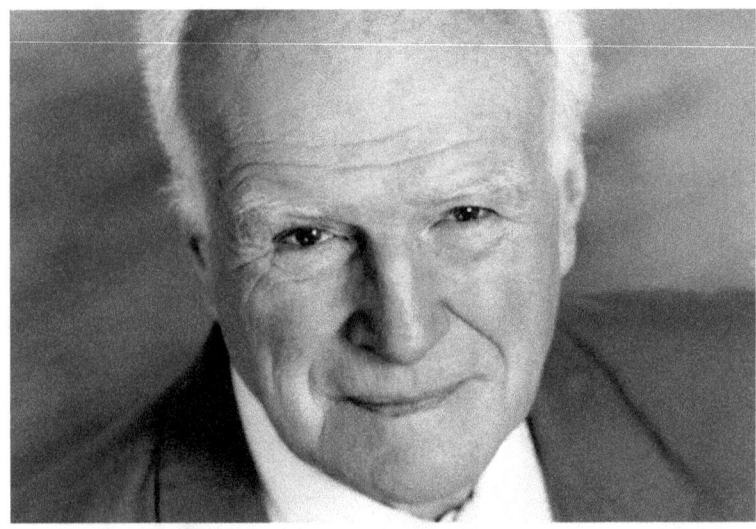

Dr. Fraser Mustard

had also been a member of Varsity Blue—the University of Toronto's collegiate football team. He and John Evans had both been tight-end teammates.

"Dr. William (Bill) Spaulding was the Outpatient Director at University of Toronto. He had supervised both Dr. Evans and Dr. Walsh during their residency. Dr. Spaulding was trained in internal medicine and psychiatry, and he was a student of medical history. He understood how to get things done and had founded many interdisciplinary programs involving social work, psychology, and public health. He had even created a diabetic day care unit. He was the most

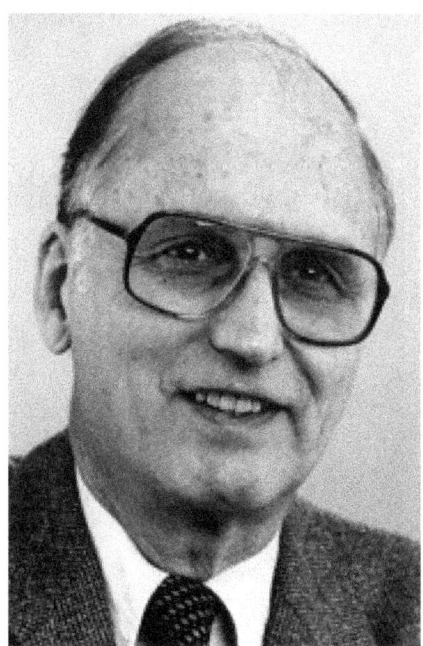

Dr. Bill Spaulding

senior, experienced member of the Founders. Dr. Bill Spaulding was an avuncular character—easily approached—and a great diagnostician too.

"Dr. Jim Anderson was a 'hip,' first-rate anatomist at the University of Toronto. He had already created the Kool School in Toronto. It was an alternative high school for marginalized young people who were different and had experienced discrimination. Some of them were the weed-smoking hippie types. The educational methods employed there were in agreement with Dr. Evans' thoughts on medical education. Dr. Jim was accepting, freewheeling, irreverent, and a jokester—with a serious side as well. He was intensely interested in the origins of humans

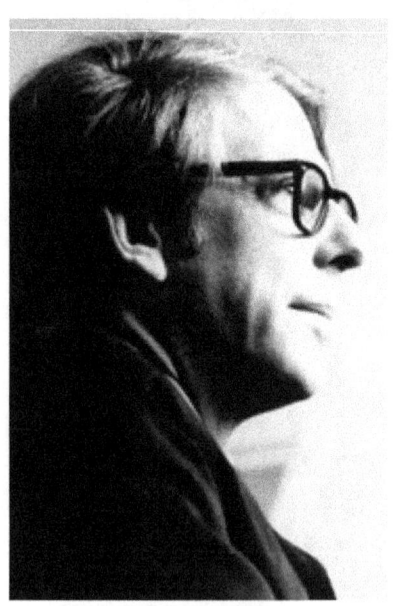

Dr. Jim Anderson

and studied archeology and anthropology. He travelled the world and had participated in many field studies.

"These very different individuals had all been magically brought together by Dr. Evans, as a result of their University of Toronto connection. Much is now known about the ingredients needed to build optimal human teams. There has to be a personality mix that includes: the visionary; the predictable practical thinker; the data-driven logical problem solver, and the intuitive one—an expert in relationships and social awareness. Perhaps it was by design, or maybe sheer luck was involved. Dr. Evans had created the perfect team. Their collective creative genius proved to be an unstoppable force as they developed a bold new curriculum. They became known as the Founding Fathers."

After glancing at my watch, I interrupted the history lesson because my tutorial group meeting was starting in less than thirty minutes—we were going to have to hustle.

"Please look straight ahead because MUMC is just coming into view. There it is—that giant block of concrete on the right. Make note of the fact that all the unsightly plumbing, mechanicals, and stairwells are on full display. They're arranged in columns up and down the exterior.

"Next, please turn your attention to the left and appreciate all the pretty Tudor homes across the street—now dwarfed by this eyesore. I wonder what's happening to property values and if many of the home owners are making plans to move."

We parked in the underground lot and walked toward a small room on the third floor, where my tutorial group was meeting. Along the way, we encountered the amazingly colorful striped carpet that welcomed everyone on the main floor, as well as sculptures, abstract paintings, and patterned concrete block walls—reminiscent of a Frank Lloyd Wright façade I'd seen in Arizona. The striking interior of the building was in sharp contrast to the ugliness of the exterior.

"Here's the Health Science Library, and just over there is the Ewart Angus Centre. As our only large lecture hall, it's where my seventy-two classmates and I meet on special occasions, such as when Sir Edmund Hillary visited. He mesmerized all of us with the account of his ascent of Mount Everest, along with his Sherpa guide. They had accomplished the feat without the assistance of supplemental oxygen.

"By the way, I'm a member of the class of 1975. We are the fourth group of students admitted to participate in this grand experiment. There is an almost even split between male and female students—unheard of at the time. And no other medical class in the world has a more diverse mix of talent: engineers, a Jesuit priest, an airline pilot, business executives, researchers and a concert pianist. There was a wide range of ages too.

"Let's stop and catch our breath, because the meeting room is just around the corner. I'll introduce you to the professor and my six classmates, and then you can take a seat along the wall. I've already arranged some chairs.

"My group will be seated at a large round table, and the focus of our discussions the past few weeks has been the heart and lungs. The module is called Pumping and Puffing. You will not be a distraction, because we often have observers from other institutions attending our sessions to see how it all works."

After the usual light-hearted banter, the professor opened a small box, emptied its contents, and read from a script.

"A fifty-eight year old obese male is your next patient. He is new to your practice and is complaining of chest pain. I'll pretend I'm the patient. What questions would you like to ask me?"

This type of questioning would never take place in traditional programs until students were in the clinical rotation of their training—the final year before graduation. However, here we were—first-year students, barely into our second month—already working with family doctors and seeing real patients.

Even if we did not know the answer, we were encouraged to problem-solve by thinking outside the box and using our imaginations.

We all chimed in and asked questions. 'How long have you had the pain; describe the discomfort; where exactly is the pain; does anything trigger your distress; does anything make it go away; how long does it last?' We even inquired about smoking and family history.

The professor asked if there were any tests we'd like to order to assist in our diagnosis and then handed me an EKG for interpretation. I'd never seen an electrocardiogram before and fumbled for a response. One of my classmates, however, had recently purchased a skinny little book called *Rapid Interpretation of EKG's* and asked to look at the long strip of paper. She applied the step-by-step approach she'd gleaned from the book and commented on rate, rhythm, and axis. Something called a Q wave was present in the inferior leads, indicating the patient likely had a heart attack in the past.

We were all stunned by her newly acquired EKG

interpretation skills, and she agreed to meet with us after the tutorial to show us the book.

A chest X-ray was then produced and placed in a view box. No one volunteered to read the film because we had no clue. We didn't even notice it had been mounted backwards. There was an awkward silence.

The preceptor then handed us some lab results that mystified us too, and the discussion and questioning lasted about an hour. In the end, we all agreed to refer this imaginary patient to a cardiologist—we suspected angina—and prescribed sublingual nitroglycerine tablets if the pain recurred. The only reason we knew about nitro was because the grandfather of one of my classmates used it for his heart pain. We concluded the problem box patient should go to the emergency room if the pill did not work.

Our next tutorial was scheduled in three days, and one member of the group volunteered to set up a brief session with a radiologist, where we all could learn how to interpret a chest X-ray.

At the start of the Pumping and Puffing module, we had all been provided with a handout that contained suggested textbooks, library-based slide tape shows, and a list of physicians and clinics we could call when in need of help. Some of us preferred to study alone, like me. Others worked best in study groups. While everything was made available, nothing was mandatory—except attending the tutorials.

The point of this novel educational approach revolved around the prediction that in the near future, there would be an explosion of new drugs, procedures, tests, and something called evidence-based trials. Physicians would not have the time to attend a lecture to remain relevant. The doctor of tomorrow would need to critically assess new information, eliminate anecdotal and unsupported treatment plans, and incorporate new protocols into their everyday patient management. McMaster was providing us with self-directed learning tools and critical assessment skills so we could stay up to date throughout our career.

The program was also demonstrating the effectiveness of working in groups, predicting that the solo practitioner model would be replaced by multi-discipline entities. In this scenario, problems would be solved by a team. Our tutorial group meetings served as the template.

Today's get-together was over, and I turned back to my guests.

"Alright, everyone, I hope you enjoyed sitting in. I'm scheduled to spend the afternoon at Dr.

Kemp's office. However, before we leave for his office, I have to visit the anatomy lab. On the way there, I want to stop at the bookstore and purchase *Rapid Interpretation of EKG's*. It looks like it is an easy and straightforward instruction manual. I walk rather quickly, so try to keep up."

The book was in stock—at less than ten dollars—quite a bargain. I couldn't wait to get back to my apartment later and read it.

"Here's the reception area for the anatomy department. You'll have to wait here because the public is not allowed inside the anatomy lab. I'll only be about fifteen minutes. Dr. Jim Anderson—one of the Founding Fathers—is expecting me. He is an anatomist, and the cadaver assigned to me and several classmates is waiting. It is wrapped in damp cloths, smells of formaldehyde, is dark brown in color, and has a leather-like texture.

"Since you can't come in, let me describe the lab for you. It's a large room that is occupied by many metal tables, some of which will be surrounded by students who are studying their cadaver. Along the walls are many shelving units stacked with big and little jars. They contain perfectly dissected body parts: brains sliced in half; hearts opened to expose the valves; kidneys; a liver; stomachs, and everything else imaginable. There is a series of tiny bottles—lined in a row—containing fetuses at various stages of development.

"There is a complete skeleton standing in a corner supported by a metal frame on wheels. The walls are adorned with drawings and charts. Countertops are loaded with microscopes and books. The entire space is white and impeccably clean—like an operating room. Everyone tends to whisper as if they are in a church. We are all aware of the generous souls who donated their bodies to assist in our learning. Respect, thanks, and reverence are words that come to mind."

After putting on a gown and gloves, I spied Dr. Anderson and introduced myself again. We'd met several times before, but there were so many new students. I explained that I saw a patient last week at Dr. Kemp's office, and the family doctor diagnosed carpal tunnel syndrome. I had never heard of such a thing and was encouraged to visit the anatomy lab and locate this structure.

Dr. Anderson grasped my cadaver's right hand and turned it palm-up. Then he pointed to the carpal bones of the wrist. "They make up the floor of this so-called tunnel," he said. "The roof is composed of a thick ligament—the flexor retinaculum. Inside this space are nine tendons that pass through and flex the fingers. The median nerve also passes through the tunnel, and it looks like a white shoelace."

He further explained that obesity, fluid retention, and overuse of the hand can reduce the space in the canal. This results in pinching of the nerve and produces the characteristic symptoms that Dr. Kemp recognized.

After hurriedly writing down the names of all the structures in a personal little book I had created, I thanked Dr. Anderson, and left the lab. My guests were patiently waiting, and I told them I was going to impress Dr. Kemp with what I'd just learned.

"It's time to head toward the clinic in Stoney Creek. However, I'm starving and am going to stop along the way at Harvey's for a burger, fries, and chocolate shake. I always ask for extra dill pickles."

No one objected—they were as hungry as me. While eating, I explained that my role at the clinic, up to this point, was to escort the patient to an exam room, record weight, measure vital signs, and ask why they were seeing the doctor today. It was an opportunity to practice my history-taking skills. After leaving the room, I'd read the chart and then report to Dr. Kemp. He preferred to be called Dr. Bob. Everything sounded simple enough, but I was having trouble.

First of all, I couldn't read his writing, and second, the charts were the most unusual things I'd ever seen. Each visit was recorded on a small index card that was subsequently inserted into a long plastic credit-card holder—the type that folds up like an accordion. I couldn't figure out how to fold and unfold the contraption—it was a Mobius strip of patient records.

For the life of me, I could not fasten the blood pressure cuff on the patient's arm correctly. The Velcro tabs would never be facing each other. And since they couldn't adhere, the cuff was completely untethered. As I inflated the bladder, the cuff would fly off the arm—startling both me and the patient.

Of course I'd apologize, turn the cuff around and reapply it, only to discover the Velcro tabs were still not facing each other. I'd try turning it backwards and then upside down. My fumbling caught the attention of the nurse, who had repeatedly demonstrated the correct application. I still couldn't figure it out.

She shook her head in exasperation, and I'm sure she reported my incompetence to Dr. Kemp.

I could already feel a growing anxiety as I finished my French fries. In a few minutes, I would have to face that perplexing blood pressure machine. Given the difficulty that I was experiencing with the foldable charts and the cuff, I had become convinced I must have some kind of neurological disorder that had robbed me of my spatial orientation abilities.

Dr. Bob and the staff appeared tense today. I hoped that it wasn't because they knew I was coming. After a rather cold reception, I was instructed to see Ricky. He was a fifteen year old boy who required a sports physical and some paperwork completed—he was trying out for the local high school basketball team.

I placed the blood pressure cuff on Ricky's arm, and, to my amazement, it fit correctly. I recorded 190/110. He was an athletic young fellow with an unremarkable past history, and I was just wrapping up my questioning when Dr. Kemp burst into the room. He appeared hurried and asked if I had finally managed to record a blood pressure. I nodded and showed Dr. Bob the quite elevated reading. He looked at me and sighed.

Assuming my measurement was erroneous, he then measured the pressure himself—190/110. Dr. Kemp switched the cuff to the right arm—190/110—listened to the heart, sat back, and appeared puzzled.

Dr. Bob left the room and returned a moment later with a much larger and wider cuff. He had the patient remove his pants and measured the pressure in the left leg, placing his stethoscope behind the knee. I didn't even know you could check the pressure in a leg.

It was 100/66.

Dr. Bob instructed me to find the patient's mother in the waiting room. Once everyone was seated, Dr. Kemp announced—using his most calming voice—that he was almost certain Ricky had coarctation of the aorta. It was the only time he had ever diagnosed this condition after forty years of practice. He explained that Ricky had been born with a narrowing of the main artery—the aorta—several inches from where it exits the heart. This had created a situation where there was a reduced blood flow to the lower part of the body, just like what would happen if you kinked a garden hose. And above the narrowing, there was excessive pressure that placed great strain on the pump, increasing the risk of heart attack and stroke.

The young fellow was completely blindsided by this news, and was especially upset to learn he could not play sports until he saw a specialist. He was likely going to require surgery.

The rest of the afternoon was quite ordinary. Dr. Kemp allowed me to have a break and supplied me with his copy of *Harrison's Principles of Internal Medicine*. It is one of the essential books that every doctor must have, and I read all about coarctation and other related congenital conditions. We never did have time to discuss carpal tunnel.

However, Dr. Bob told me he was pleased I had figured out the blood pressure machine and was impressed at how quickly I was learning. Next week, he wanted to take me to the hospital where we would make rounds together. I was thrilled.

"So there you have it. You've just experienced what it's like to be a medical student, albeit for only a few hours. It's time for me to drive you back to downtown Hamilton where we met this morning. You've had quite a long day and obviously enjoyed tagging along.

"As for me, I still have a few hours of work ahead. I'm going to grab some food and read my new EKG book. And then I want to add today's new pearls of important facts to my little reference book. I can't wait to tell my tutorial group about coarctation and its treatment. Talk soon."

The Doctor Is In

CHAPTER FIVE
MY FRESHMAN YEAR

The first year of any medical school program is hard enough. It appears that I had to add to this challenge by getting married, adopting a beagle, competing on the varsity golf team, and secretly cross-dressing. And I did it all with no reliable source of income!

On looking back at my decision-making during this time, I now realize more clearly why I did not receive the Einstein award—the brightest bulb trophy—during my freshman year. There was always next time.

My wedding to Mary Jo took place on December 14, 1972. I was completing my fourth month of medical school, and she was enrolled in a diploma nursing program at St. Joseph's Hospital. We were both twenty-two years old, madly in love, and had almost no savings in the bank. At least she could work at a summer job. I was in a program with no breaks, and my previous summer job earnings were quickly being depleted. We heard comments that suggested we were too young to marry, and it would never work out. Of course we were not listening.

The wedding was quite the event, because her parents were well-to-do and Mary Jo was their only daughter. The guest list exceeded 250, the reception was at the Hamilton Golf and Country Club, everything was decorated for Christmas, it was snowing, my parents made the treacherous five hour journey from Ottawa, and Mary Jo's mother smelled like a fish. Let me explain.

Her dress had been created at the home of a talented seamstress. It was hanging in a hallway, waiting to be delivered the next day. That evening, the dressmaker cooked salmon for dinner, and the odor permeated every thread of the magnificent gown that was only a few feet away from the kitchen.

The odor was not noticed initially, but as my new mother-in-law warmed the garment, especially during the dancing part of the evening, everyone looked for the source of the fishy intrusion. The search finally ended at her feet, and no amount of perfume could banish that salmon from the room.

We received a honeymoon gift of a trip to Hawaii, along with dishes, a toaster, tea cups, silver serving trays, cutlery, and so much more. However, none of this helped pay our rent.

A classmate, Tom, mentioned to me how he was making a little extra money. First, a researcher needed volunteers to test some new endoscopy equipment that he was developing. I was paid fifty dollars for allowing this scientist to pass a scope down my throat and into my stomach. It was the most horrible thirty minutes of my life, and I declined his offer to volunteer again.

The second job paid quite well too, and was much more pleasurable. The infertility clinic was looking for sperm donors, and Tom and I donated whenever they called. The required self-stimulation married quite well with the self-directed learning that served as the mainstay of the medical program.

However, this was no way to support a new wife. How could I answer the probing question of my father-in-law, "Tell me, son, exactly what are you doing to make ends meet?" I replied that it was hard, but I was working on it. Of course he did not understand the double entendre.

I had to find a better way to pay the bills. Some of my classmates came from wealthy families and did not share my dilemma. Many others were taking out student loans, but my father cautioned me about borrowing money. Several others had enlisted in the Canadian Armed Forces—the Medical Officer's Training Program. This MOTP initiative provided the participant with a rank—second lieutenant—and a handsome salary.

Of course there was a catch. The enrollee had to complete a modified basic training, report to the base at Downsview in Toronto every few months, and serve for a minimum of two years after graduation. Dad thought this was a terrific idea, especially since he was a World War II veteran—a US paratrooper and drill sergeant.

Mary Jo and I weighed our options. We were tired of being broke; I was fearful that most of Hamilton would eventually look like me if I continued working for the infertility clinic, and we liked the sound of an adventure. I made a few phone calls and enlisted early in the New Year.

This was a happy time in our life. Of course we studied diligently while listening to the Carpenters. Their big hit was "Close to You," and it became our song. I think every young couple has a song they identify with—a tune that perfectly captures the moment that something mysterious called love takes root.

We welcomed a rescue dog into our home—Laddy—an energetic beagle. He was an escape artist, and we got used to walking the streets every time he eloped. It was an unusual way to meet our neighbors, and we were all mystified by Laddy's lack of a homing instinct. If allowed, he would have followed his nose to the end of the earth. He ate off our plates if we became distracted for even a second, and usually went potty inside the house.

There were camping trips, too, and Mary Jo pursued hobbies including knitting, macramé, painting, and creating stained glass window art. I played just enough golf to win several tournaments and captain the McMaster varsity golf team to two OUAA championships.

The end of the day was our time to share stories. Mary Jo had many nursing encounters to report, and my medical school adventures continued too. I remember telling her about a tutorial group visit to an inpatient facility for disabled children. Many of these young people had been abandoned by their parents. The only family they really had was the staff at the center.

Their appearances shook me to my core. I saw children with heads the size of pumpkins due to untreated hydrocephaly, and a young male with Lesch-Nyhan syndrome—wearing a helmet and restraints—in an effort to protect him from self-mutilation. His lips and part of his tongue were missing because of his compulsive biting, and every tooth had been mercifully removed. I also observed cases of uncontrollable ataxia, shaking and writhing caused by: cerebral palsy, Huntington's chorea, and Friedreich's ataxia.

We were there to learn about abnormal physical signs during our neurology module. It was a jaw-dropping experience. I was most touched by the tender care being provided by the dedicated staff members. It was another manifestation of love, and I felt very small in their presence.

There was something else I engaged in when I had a rare moment alone. I cross-dressed and dreamed of being Bobbi. I just wanted to live life as my true and authentic self.

I shared this part of me with Mary Jo, and she reluctantly accepted my behavior. She even used her considerable sewing talents, and made several female outfits for me. Mary Jo made it clear that no one else—especially her family—was ever to find out about this. Of course I was appreciative. However, I felt ashamed as I sneaked around like a criminal. Without her knowing, I occasionally ventured outside to experience the world as a woman. And then I would be gripped by intense fear. What if someone recognized me? What if I had a flat tire or got stopped by the police? I would race home—breathless—and quickly change before anyone knocked on the door.

This closeted behavior was gradually eroding my self-confidence. At times I sensed that my professors, classmates, or spectators at a golf tournament could see right through me. My sinfulness was readily apparent, or so I thought. I did what I could to be invisible and shied away from the spotlight.

Crying was often involved, and a constant sadness enveloped me. I had to stay busy and deprive myself of any time to think. I felt trapped.

The Doctor Is In

CHAPTER SIX
EARLY EXPERIENCES

We moved into an apartment that did not allow pets. Laddy found a home with a beagle-loving owner, and I remember celebrating his departure that evening. Two of our new high-rise neighbors were Bart and his wife. Bart was a fellow classmate, and we became fast friends. We shared experiences and stories, although I don't believe we were ever in the same tutorial group together. Of course I had to tell him about my coarctation patient and the hospital rounds I made with Dr. Kemp.

Dr. Bob was absolutely worshiped by patients and healthcare workers alike. I could only dream of earning similar respect from my community somewhere in the future.

Aside from endlessly reading textbooks and viewing slide tape shows, I signed up for extra experiences. As an example, I accompanied a police officer for an entire shift and observed him mediate a family dispute, calm the drivers involved in a minor fender bender, and call for support to rescue an unconscious homeless person in Gore Park.

I volunteered to shadow an emergency room doctor one evening at Saint Joseph's Hospital.

He instructed me to see a fifteen-year-old girl with abdominal pain and report back to him. I remember parting the curtain and introducing myself to a somewhat chubby young lady and her mother. The cramping had started earlier in the day, and it came and went—involving her entire lower abdomen. There was no nausea, diarrhea, fever, chills, or painful urination. I had been prepared to diagnose appendicitis, but her symptoms did not match up.

The nurse showed me her vital signs—normal—as I placed my inexperienced hand on her ample tummy. The swelling was unmistakable, even for a rookie. The girl was pregnant… and in labor, no less!

I quickly excused myself and tracked down the emergency room physician. He listened to my story, dropped what he was doing, and rushed to her room. He performed a vaginal exam, and, to everyone's surprise, she was fully dilated and pushing. The delivery was imminent.

The doctor directed the staff to call labor and delivery—stat—and prepare them to receive the patient. Between contractions, the daughter and mother argued.

The young lady was peppered with questions.

"How could this have happened? Who is the

father? Is it that good-for-nothing little creep you've been hanging around with? Why didn't you tell me about this?"

Her father appeared suddenly—in the middle of another prolonged contraction—spewing angry words like *disappointed, shameful,* and *sinful.*

I'd heard enough and told the parents to shut up. They could carry on their conversation later because, at the moment, we had an obstetrical emergency on our hands. We all had to pitch in and help their daughter.

I ran after the gurney as she was whisked away to the Labor and Delivery floor. What a mess! Unknown due date, no prenatal care, and she had been starving to hide the growing new life from the world's prying eyes.

Standing on my tiptoes, I watched her push the new little boy into his uncertain future. Her parents resumed arguing, the baby was growth retarded, and the exhausted young mother was crying. Could this really be happening?

Returning to the emergency room, I saw several more routine patients and then retreated to my car. My head was full of unanswerable questions. What would happen to that precious newborn? Would he die? Maybe he'd be disabled. Perhaps he might be adopted out. Or possibly he'd live with the young mother and her family. How would this change the trajectory of her life? Did the biological father know about the pregnancy, and was he contemplating stepping forward?

Until starting my training, I had no idea about the complicated lives unfolding all around me. There were so many issues, and I felt overwhelmed. Where does one start?

CHAPTER SEVEN
CLERKSHIP—CARE FOR A SMOKE?

The first two years of the program flew by. Mary Jo had completed her nursing program and was working in the operating room at St. Joseph's Hospital. My knowledge base was now quite impressive.

From time to time I met with my mentor, Dr. McAuley. We discussed my anxiety about how I was doing. Was I keeping up with my classmates? Were there core areas of study I had missed that would come back to haunt me?

Without exams, there was no measuring stick. I never felt like I had finished an assignment or completed a curriculum item because there was no definite beginning or end to a module. The entire program felt nebulous—a self-directed mess—unique to the individual student. And I wasn't the only one who was experiencing this tension. Many of my classmates were struggling with the same uncertainties too.

Of course, Dr. Ron reassured me that my subjective evaluations from every preceptor were great. However, I had been brought up on exams. In a year, I would have to sit for the big license examination—independent from the medical school. I know it sounds ridiculous, but

I would have given anything for the occasional test along the way.

The clerkship had begun—my final year of medical school. The focus was mainly clinical. As a clerk, I was immersed full-time in every major hospital department for a few weeks: emergency, psychiatry, labor and delivery, surgery, pediatrics, and internal medicine. I wore a short white coat—the long ones were reserved for real doctors. I carried the stethoscope my parents had given me along with a reflex hammer in my right pocket, and a copy of the *Washington Manual of Medical Therapeutics* in my left.

Aside from my hospital-based duties, I still met weekly with yet another tutorial group where we discussed various topics.

In this third and final year, the expectations and responsibilities ramped up immediately. I was no longer an observer. Chief residents, senior staff and attending physicians were now asking pointed questions, assigning many chores, and watching my every move. Their criticisms were often scathing and sarcastic. You never knew when you might be singled out.

I disliked being watched. It unnerved me. I feared someone would finally discover that I was not that bright. Even worse, perhaps my secret might be uncovered—my sin. Hiding was like a cloak-

and-dagger game, and my guilty conscious was the end result.

Even though I was low on the totem pole, I was now an important part of the team and required to stay in the hospital—on call—every four nights or so.

***

My initial rotation was obstetrics, and the ward was quiet on that first morning. The chief resident showed me to a room containing several plastic models. One was the skeleton of a female pelvis that highlighted all the bony landmarks used to measure the progress of labor. The other was a replica of a baby's skull. I practiced placing two fingers inside the pelvis, with my eyes closed, and tried to identify the bony protrusions.

At the same time, I passed the tiny head into the pelvis and observed how the skull rotated as it passed through the birth canal. I memorized the pattern on the skull that was created by the soft spots—the fontanelles—and the intersecting bones that were not yet fused. The recognition of these landmarks was crucial. It was the only way to know if the baby was oriented correctly or facing the wrong way, which would spell trouble during labor.

Later, as I emerged from the classroom, a woman

exited the elevator—her husband in tow—and presented herself at the nurses' station. She appeared to be in considerable distress and was escorted immediately to a labor room.

Several minutes later the L&D nurse summoned the resident to the room, and I tagged along. This was the patient's first pregnancy. She was several days over-due, and contractions had started around midnight. Her water broke in the car on the way to the hospital.

After introducing ourselves, the resident asked me to examine the patient and see how far along her labor had progressed. I nervously placed my right hand into an examination glove, sprayed my second and third gloved digits with an antiseptic solution, and tentatively inserted my probing fingers. Her vagina felt nothing like the plastic model, and I couldn't identify a single landmark. I pushed forward as far as my long fingers would extend and bumped into a hard object—a head?

And then quite abruptly, my index finger was grasped. Startled, I abruptly removed my hand from the vagina. The resident looked surprised, took me aside and quietly asked, "What the f*** was that all about?"

I whispered that something had grabbed me and wouldn't let go. He looked at me in disbelief, dismissively pushed me aside, smiled at the patient, and examined her for himself. A look of concern quickly occupied his face.

The resident instructed the nurse to apply a fetal monitor, start an intravenous and page the patient's obstetrician—stat. Then he turned his attention to the expectant parents and calmly explained the problem. Their baby's head was coming down the birth canal appropriately. However, an arm and hand were accompanying the head, and it would be impossible to deliver the baby vaginally given this abnormal presentation. The resident further explained that the extra space created by the hand could allow the cord to sneak by—a prolapse—and jeopardize the baby's life. At the moment, their child was in great condition. The prudent course of action was a Cesarean section.

Now I understood what had happened. My probing finger had touched the baby's palm and had triggered a grasp reflex. Those little fingers had held me tight for a moment and caused me to startle.

The anxious young couple was relieved to hear that their obstetrician had just arrived. The findings were confirmed, a C-section performed, and there was jubilation everywhere.

When it was all over, I reflected on the resident's performance: he recognized a potentially serious problem and took charge; instituted emergency measures; appeared calm under pressure; reassured the patient, and demonstrated obvious surgical skills while assisting the obstetrician. There was a lot to digest and internalize.

Later that night, I participated in an absolutely routine delivery. Standing at the foot of the table, between the wide-spread legs of an expectant mother, I exhorted her to push harder. I was astounded by the endurance required to deliver a baby. I had observed athletes engaged in peak performance—I was an athlete—and nothing I'd ever seen approached the raw, animal-like effort required of a mother at this moment.

The baby was extruded—inch by inch—into my waiting hands. I was alarmed at how slippery the squirming pink cherub was—covered in amniotic fluid and vernix. I'd heard of a family doctor who fumbled a baby at this very hospital just a few years earlier. It landed on its head and died a short time later. I held on tight.

This delivery was my first—a moment I will never forget. I completed my on-call night, attended a gynecology clinic the next day, and then finally returned to the apartment and Mary Jo. I couldn't stop talking about the miracle I'd been part of. And then I collapsed into bed, exhausted.

I delivered several more babies during that

rotation. What scared me the most were the forceps that the obstetricians skillfully wielded while extracting a stuck newborn from the birth canal. They looked like sleek and shiny weapons of war.

The last delivery I attended during clerkship involved a first-time mother and a marathon labor. An epidural was in place. By two in the morning, the head was barely visible and she was exhausted. I was being supervised by the Chief of Obstetrics—a ruggedly handsome man with close cropped curly hair, and big hands and feet. He looked haggard as he sat on the stool next to me—lighted cigarette in hand!

This fact in itself is hard to believe, but in the summer of 1974, personnel smoked everywhere in the hospital. I personally witnessed coronary-care unit staff smoking at the nurses' station, while they watched the cardiac monitors of cigarette-ravaged heart attack patients.

The obstetrician placed his smoke on the edge of a countertop, stood up, donned a glove, and examined the patient. He announced that forceps were required and asked which type I wanted to use. What he didn't realize was that I didn't want to use Simpsons, Tuckers, Kielands, or Pipers. I simply wanted to run out the door right away and hide.

He chose a pair of gleaming Simpsons and handed me the left one. I introduced it ever so cautiously into the birth canal and then followed with the right. The two shafts articulated perfectly, and I locked them together. He checked to be sure everything was positioned correctly, plopped back down on his stool and resumed puffing. I waited for a contraction, cued the patient to push—she was numb from the waist down—and I gently pulled.

The Chief gestured for me to pull in a more downward direction—the cigarette serving as a pointer for added drama! At just the right moment, he told me to pull upward. My goodness! The head was right there! I removed the blades, and the baby followed into my waiting arms. My scrubs were drenched in sweat. The ordeal was over, except for the sewing, because there was quite a sizeable vaginal tear.

***

I had the weekend off before starting my next rotation—psychiatry—and I needed a break. I went to Chedoke Civic Golf Course, where I had worked a few summers before. My plan was to hit some balls at the practice range. Back then, every accomplished golfer had a shag bag full of golf balls, all marked with a personal symbol as a statement of ownership. After hitting balls onto the range, I'd wait for other golfers to finish, and then we'd walk together to collect our personalized balls. Mine were usually in a neat little cluster because I could aim really well.

While waiting, I struck up a conversation with Bob—a good player—and a friend. He was a handsome fellow, strong as a bull, and looked more like a football player than a golfer. He was regaling me with a story about a great shot he had recently struck in a tournament, when I suddenly heard a loud sound. It startled me. Had there been a car accident?

And then I realized Bob had been hit in the head by an errant tee shot from the tenth tee—that same tenth tee where Mr. Turnbull had died from a heart attack years ago, while I stood by and did nothing. Bob stood in place—motionless—his story interrupted as the ball bounced away. And then he began to topple toward me. I caught him, slowed his descent to the ground, and we both went down in a heap. He was out cold as he lay on his back. I scrambled to my feet while other golfers approached to stop and stare.

Taking command of the situation, I ordered one of the onlookers to run to the pro-shop and call an ambulance. While I was checking his vital signs, Bob began to twitch and had what appeared to be a seizure for a few seconds. I'd read that head-injured patients often vomit, so I rolled him on his side in anticipation of that occurrence. I didn't want him to aspirate the vomitus. He was still unconscious when the ambulance arrived.

I informed the paramedics of the circumstances surrounding the injury, and they whisked Bob away. Then I collected his golf balls and clubs and brought them to the pro shop, where they would await his hoped-for return.

As it turned out, Bob made a full recovery and we joked about the event when we met later in life. However, that incident made me realize I was making great strides toward becoming a doctor. I was not just a Good Samaritan or even a kind person. My knowledge and training were now allowing me to help in even more meaningful ways.

This was a powerful feeling.

CHAPTER EIGHT
NO THANKS, DR FREUD

The receptionist at the Hamilton Psychiatric Hospital smiled and directed me to the office of my preceptor—an esteemed psychiatrist. His resident, an intern and several other members of the team were already assembled. Ward rounds were about to begin. I was starting my rotation in psychiatry.

The hospital was to the west of a main thoroughfare in Hamilton that I had driven by many times over the years. It was a place that was shrouded in mystery: my father and the rest of the community called it the "Nut House." I was more than a little nervous.

We entered a ward, through locked doors, and proceeded to walk from room to room—pushing a cart filled with patient charts and order forms in front of the entourage.

I couldn't help but notice the patients in the hallway: their expressionless faces, the shuffling gaits, drooling mouths. They looked like zombies. I wondered what behaviors they had exhibited that warranted this kind of chemical restraint. Although I said nothing, the place felt dangerous to me.

This was my least favorite rotation. I met the strangest people. One middle-aged woman told me that she was famous and had invented the Nautilus submarine. Another told me she was from a faraway planet called Etherea, and made frequent trips back and forth. Several claimed the police and the military were trying to find and kill them. Another male talked non-stop for hours. I couldn't follow even a single thread of what he was talking about.

Of course not all the stories were this dramatic. In the outpatient clinic, I observed many patients who were struggling with depression, obsessions, neurosis, hypochondriasis, and phobias.

There were discussions on delirium, psychosis, dementia, mood disorders, and schizophrenia, as well as their diagnosis and treatment. Psychoanalysis and the Freudian theories about libido, the id, ego, superego, and the power of the unconscious mind sounded like a lot of mumbojumbo—at least to me. Even though there were no objective tests, tricyclic antidepressants, MAO inhibitors, tranquilizers, electro-convulsive therapy, and anti-psychotics were all liberally prescribed.

I learned here that individuals like me, who cross-dressed, were thought to be afflicted with a psychiatric illness. This only added to my discomfort. At least this rotation afforded me access to many psychiatry and psychology journals. During some free time, I'd surreptitiously look for papers about transsexuals and transvestites to learn more about these conditions. Time after time I would find a reference, locate the journal, open to the page of the article, and find it had been ripped out from the binding!

What was going on here? Was someone trying to prevent information like this from being distributed to the public? Or was there an individual —a doctor no less—who was trying to learn more about themselves and did not want to be discovered reading the article publically. Perhaps they desired to read it in the privacy of their own home, where no one would discover their secret.

I sensed that I was not alone. There was another troubled cross-dresser working in that hospital. If the poor soul was a Catholic, at least I would have company in hell.

***

During this psychiatry rotation, my weekly tutorial group met for several sessions with one of the most interesting persons I'd ever met—Dr. David Sackett.

A large man with a full gray beard, Dr. Sackett spoke softly with a precise, measured cadence.

He was an epidemiologist and talked of double-blind randomized trials, incidence, prevalence, sensitivity, specificity, and false positives and negatives. He was an intellectual—the father of evidence-based medicine. My time with Dr. Sackett was mind-blowing. And then I had to return to the specialty of psychiatry—with a straight face—and play along with its non-evidenced-based framework and treatment protocols.

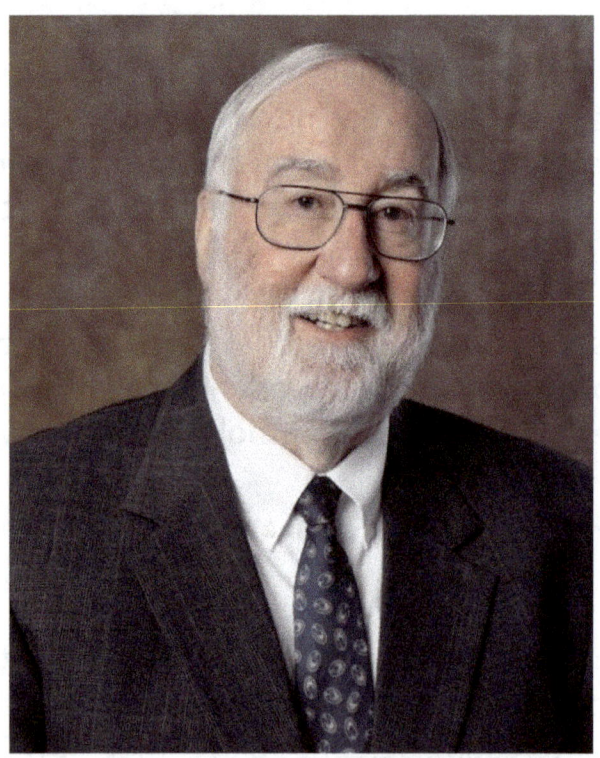

Dr. David Sackett

As I've already pointed out, this was a difficult rotation for me on many levels. However, it was not all wasted time. I learned how to better assess suicide risk, and this would allow me to intervene and possibly save a life in the future. Therapies such as supportive psychotherapy and something new called *cognitive behavioral therapy* made sense, and were supported by good studies too.

One thing was perfectly clear: I was not going to pursue a career in psychiatry.

The Doctor Is In

CHAPTER NINE
NOT READY FOR PRIME TIME

The stars had aligned and a personal meltdown was about to occur. I remember feeling sad after my psychiatry rotation. Was depression perhaps contagious?

Surgery was the next rotation, and I'd been assigned to a notoriously arrogant preceptor. Dr. Nugent had a temper and a reputation for exhibiting boorish behavior. He had several well-deserved nicknames that don't belong in this book. Guess who would be his new foil?

He rode me without mercy, delivering insulting comments on a daily basis. My presentations at rounds were admittedly uneven and, at times, disorganized. I definitely did not like surgery and often felt faint in the operating room—scrubbing out on several occasions. I'd barely make it to the change room where I'd recline on an old couch—my feet elevated higher than my head—until the light-headed feeling passed. By then I was drenched in sweat. On two occasions I actually vomited while struggling to maintain consciousness.

"You are lazy, unprepared, ignorant, and a disgrace." I heard it over and over.

While this was going on, my weekly tutorial group was given a new exercise. One by one, we were asked to assess, examine, and diagnose a programmed patient—an actor—in front of a one-way mirror. The rest of the group, along with a professor, sat behind the mirror scoring the performance. We were not given the presenting complaint ahead of time. Each evaluation took about forty-five minutes, allowing for the assessments of two classmates each week.

The thought of being stared at by my peers, the possibility of not knowing anything about the condition, and the chance that I might perform poorly were all frightening prospects. I was terrified of being humiliated.

I manipulated the schedule so that I would be the seventh and last student. To date, everyone had performed adequately, and two were really exceptional. The dreaded moment arrived and my heart was pounding—my mind went blank too. I refused to go to the monitored room where the patient was waiting. The preceptor issued a stern command. I gripped my seat, and refused to budge. One of the students attempted to pull me up from the chair. I resisted like some fearful child not wanting to attend the first day of school.

Perhaps I should have talked to Dr. McAuley or the preceptor about my difficulty with this exercise.

There might have been some accommodation arranged. However, it was too late to ask for a time-out, and my life was about to change.

Everything happened quickly. I jumped up from the chair and bolted for the door—like a trapped animal. I yelled, "I'm not going to do this!" And then I raced down the hall and out the building—wide-eyed from panic—like a crazy person. Once outside, I ran as fast as I could for about a hundred yards until I was breathless. I was running from something. However, I wasn't at all certain what it was.

I'm getting ahead of myself. This was not the last time I would run from a situation, and it was not until I was in my sixties that a psychologist helped me figure it out. After listening to my exhaustive history, he became intensely interested in the four times during my formative years where I had been the recipient of a very public shaming and humiliation. Individually, he called them small traumatic events. However, when repetitiously added together, they represented one huge trauma. He diagnosed me with post-traumatic stress syndrome—PTSD. When placed in a similar situation, reminiscent of the original events, I would be triggered. My primitive reptilian brain—the amygdala—took over and I would find myself in an existential situation. It was either fight or flight. My rational brain had been hijacked.

And I always chose to run.

This explanation made sense to me. I would not say that I have been cured. But his lessons around situational awareness, behavioral therapy and EMDR have all helped me live a less drama-filled life.

I wish I had known about this PTSD stuff during my clerkship, as it would have made all the difference. However, I was young and thought I didn't need help from anyone. This train wreck was getting ready to happen.

***

Following this awful moment, I quickly made up my mind. I was quitting the program. To hell with it! Who was I trying to fool that a cross-dressing sinner was actually worthy of becoming a physician. And maybe Dr. Nugent was right—I wasn't smart enough.

By the time I arrived home, I had calmed down considerably and explained to Mary Jo that I wanted to explore another career—professional golf—and that I was abandoning my medical studies. While she had known about my ambivalence for a long time, she hoped I would change my mind in the morning.

Actually, I wasn't sure I wanted to be a golfer,

either, but at least it gave me the appearance of having a plan.

At first, it was such a relief to be removed from the pressure cooker! I composed a letter of resignation to the dean—Dr. Fraser Mustard—and mailed it the very next day. Dr. Nugent, my surgical preceptor, received a copy and summoned me to his office at McMaster. I endured an extremely uncomfortable diatribe in which he made it clear that he considered me a typical spoiled brat from a wealthy family—selfish to the core—who couldn't stand hard work. He must have been talking about someone else because that certainly wasn't a description of my background. However, he was agitated, and I wasn't going to stand in his way.

Dr. Nugent went on to say that I should be ashamed I had wasted taxpayer dollars, while robbing another, more worthy candidate of a coveted place in the program. He thought that trading a medical career for a frivolous job in the golf business was disgraceful. If he was trying to guilt me into staying, his red-faced belligerence was having the opposite effect.

I'd heard enough, got up to leave, thanked him for his time and walked out the door—hopeful that I'd never see him again.

Then, Dr. McAuley called, and we arranged to

meet. He was concerned and asked what was going on. "Are you alright?" he asked. I explained that medicine was not for me and never had been my first choice. I told him I wanted to pursue a career in golf. He didn't buy it.

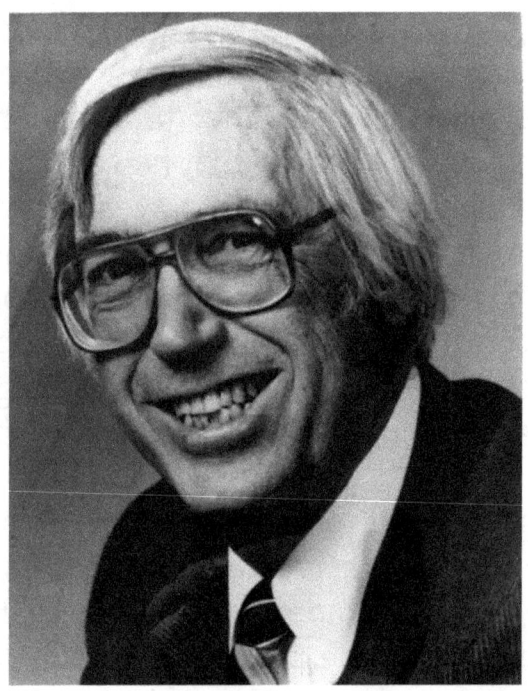

Dr. Ron McAuley

He had my original letter addressed to the dean in his hand and tore it in two pieces, saying he was not going to let me quit. The gesture startled me.

Dr. McAuley then proceeded to tell me that, in his opinion, I was going to be one of the most outstanding doctors he had ever met. He believed in me way more than I believed in myself.

Instead of letting me resign from the program, he asked if I would consider simply asking for a leave of absence. I was not enthused about this approach. I'd already told my parents, the in-laws, and a few close friends that I had quit, because I really felt certain about the decision.

In the end, however, I agreed to ask for a leave—it kept all options open—and promised to stay in touch with Dr. McAuley.

The Doctor Is In

CHAPTER TEN
LOST BUT NOT FORGOTTEN

For the first time in memory, I did not have to attend school. I no longer had to be an A student—number one in the class. The burden had been removed, albeit in a messy way. My parents were shocked but still supportive. However, my in-laws wouldn't speak to me. For them it was proof-positive that their daughter should never have married 'down' when she married me. Mary Jo's mother, in particular, had openly not liked me from the start, and I sensed she placed considerable unspoken pressure on her daughter to leave me. After all, there were so many more socially acceptable boys to date and remarry.

Winter was just around the corner, and the golf season was over. The Canadian Armed Forces wanted their subsidization money back, and they honorably discharged me. I had to find work. I sold men's clothes at the Right House and planned my tournament schedule for the next year.

We stayed committed to our wedding vows and muddled through. In fact, we tried to have a baby, only to discover Mary Jo had an infertility problem—polycystic ovaries. She would become pregnant and then miscarry repeatedly. Each of these events was devastating.

Spring arrived. I found work in the pro shop at Chedoke, and I competed as if my life depended on the results. I qualified for both provincial and national championships and found myself in contention at times. Once in the spotlight, my lack of self-belief revealed itself every time. In the middle of battle, I'd worry about my appearance or what I'd say in my victory speech. Thoughts entered my head that I might miss the ball completely or hit into the very next water hazard. My head became full of nonsensical fears.

Predictably, I would lose focus, hit errant shots, make some course management errors, and slide back into the pack. In lower profile tournaments against less skilled players, I could win. However, on the big stage I'd choke. It was very frustrating, and I didn't have a clue how to change my thinking.

As if it had been planned, Dr. McAuley called at one of those frustrating moments. "You haven't called me," he said. "What are you up to? Are you ready to come back to the program?"

I apologized for not calling. It had been rude of me. And then I reminded him I was in the golf business now and had no intention of returning. Dr. McAuley wished me well and made me promise to stay in touch. This man was not giving up on me.

***

The Doctor Is In

Winter was approaching again, and I heard of a job that paid handsomely. I became a driver for Yellow Cab—car number 105. The tips were great, and I was making a lot more in a cab than I did on the golf course.

After a few weeks, I developed a reputation for being patient and kind. The dispatcher received special requests from customers who were not used to being treated so well by a cabby. They were usually old people who moved slowly, used walkers that required placement in the trunk, took short trips, and generally tipped poorly. These fares represented a cab driver's nightmare. However, for me, they were like the old couple I had raked leaves for when I was a youngster. And they had interesting stories. They tipped me very well, especially after I carried their groceries into their homes and helped them up the steps.

By chance I was called to transport a disabled child from her home to daycare. I carried the young girl from the porch to the back seat of the cab, secured the seatbelt, loaded the wheelchair in the trunk, and sang songs with her on the way to the facility. Apparently the news of my performance spread quickly through the close-knit community of parents with similarly disabled children. I became the preferred driver for all of their loved ones. I was excelling at being a cabbie, and I loved those kids. These regular customers showered me with praise and tips.

At times, I would pick up a fare in downtown Hamilton or at the airport, only to discover it was one of my old medical professors. I avoided eye contact and conversation in the hope that this person would not recognize me. I was filled with shame.

Before long, springtime was approaching, and along with it came new hope for a more successful competitive season. I continued to drive a cab while I polished my golf game. I really didn't have a clue about the steps needed to become a professional player. I'd never had a coach, my equipment was inferior, and I could barely afford entry fees.

Not unexpectedly, my tournament play was a repeat of last year and the year before that, too. In a blink, the Canadian golf season came to a close, and I had not experienced a breakthrough moment. I was back behind the wheel of cab number 105 and driving full-time again.

One day, there was a chill in the air that discouraged potential customers from being out and about. I had pulled into a station—fifth in line for a fare—and had been waiting an hour. It was a windy autumn afternoon and multi-colored leaves swirled around the car, as if in search of a safe harbor.

This moment afforded me time to think. I'd been

out of school for almost two years and hadn't kept in touch with Dr. McAuley. My plans related to the golf business were vague and going nowhere. And there weren't any other career options that had magically appeared.

I reflected on all the jobs I'd had to date. As a youngster, I'd worked on my grandfather's farm, delivered newspapers and caddied. One summer when I was sixteen, I'd won a McMaster summer studentship and worked for a professor in his microbiology lab. I'd bagged groceries at a food store, performed backbreaking work as a laborer for the Hamilton Streets and Sanitation Department, sold men's clothes in a department store, and worked at the local golf course. And now I was a cab driver.

All of these jobs had taught me how hard the average person works to make a dollar. I knew what it felt like to be down to the last penny before every payday. I also witnessed the satisfaction that many of my blue collar co-workers derived from doing a good job, me included. Perhaps this was where my future would be.

The four cabs ahead of me had not moved, and I became nostalgic—perhaps melancholic is a better choice of words. I missed my classmates, some of my professors, my books, and the excitement of being part of something special.

Helping people was what I missed most of all.

The search for something meaningful had left me pretty beat up, and it suddenly dawned on me that the answer to my tomorrow was hiding in plain sight. I had to call Dr. McAuley and talk with him right away. After returning home, I scrambled to find his contact information.

He had gone for the day, so I left a message.

"Hello, Dr. Ron. It's Bob. Bob Lancaster. I hope you're well. I'd like to talk to you about something. Please give me a call as soon as you can. Bye for now."

CHAPTER ELEVEN
A SECOND CHANCE

Dr. McAuley listened to my message when he arrived at work the next morning. The only number he knew to call was my home phone, and I was already at work. Remember, this was 1976, and well before the invention of emails, cell phones, and texts.

I had several interesting customers that day and even snagged a lucrative trip to the airport in Toronto. Perhaps this was going to be my lucky day.

Finally home, I was counting my earnings while Mary Jo prepared dinner. The phone rang and I ran to pick it up. I fumbled the receiver, and it fell to the floor. I became tangled in the cord as I said, "Hello."

"Hello Bob. It's Dr. McAuley. I haven't heard from you in a long time. Are you alright, and how is Mary Jo?"

"We're both doing well, and it's great to hear your voice. Dr. McAuley, I need your help. I want to come back to school. Do you know what procedure I have to follow?"

Dr. Ron was overjoyed. He said this was the best

news he'd heard in a long time. He wanted to know what had happened to change my mind.

There were so many reasons, and I didn't know where to start. On looking back, I had been twenty-one years old when I was accepted into the program—immature and naïve. Now I was twenty-six. During the past five years I had married; assumed the responsibilities that come with being a spouse; supported Mary Jo through her miscarriages and the sadness that remained; failed at my golfing dreams; worked at several jobs and met many people who were different than me. I also realized I missed helping people in a really meaningful way, and that I was wasting my natural caregiving talents. There were patients who needed my assistance now and for years to come.

Dr. McAuley was silent—had the connection been lost?

When he finally spoke, Dr. Ron's voice diminished to a whisper, and it was wrapped in sadness.

"Bob, your leave of absence expired a year ago. You can't simply jump back into the program like nothing happened. You're going to have to reapply for admission—along with the other four thousand new applicants—and hopefully be accepted again. I am so sorry."

I was stunned—at a loss for words—and then blurted out, "Oh my goodness! What have I done?"

Dr. McAuley broke the silence. "Bob, I'll see what I can do. Give me a few days. I'll call you back."

He ended the call, and I didn't know what to do except… cry… and keep driving and groveling for tips. The deadline for medical school applications had already passed, and I would have to wait another year before reapplying. It was too late to apply for graduate school, so even starting a career in biology would be delayed. I would need to come up with a new plan because continuing to be a cabby had become mind-numbing.

As promised, Dr. McAuley called back about a week later and had some news. He did not waste any time.

"Bob, I got you back in."

"Dr. McAuley, would you please repeat that? I want to be sure I heard you correctly."

"I got you back in. You'll be hearing from the director of the program soon. A plan will be developed to transition you back into clerkship. Congratulations! I'm so happy for you and Mary Jo."

Of course, this was a life changing moment for me. I had no idea what Dr. McAuley must have done to win my reinstatement. There was no way to adequately thank him.

At this point, everything moved quickly. The owner of the cab was sad to see me leave. The dispatcher said he had no idea who he would find to transport the special-needs children to and from their programs. I didn't know any other drivers because we worked in isolation, so there was no one else to bid farewell.

After meeting with the program director, it was decided that I should repeat several modules from the first two years of the program. They had been significantly updated since I last finished them. I was inserted into the class of 1978 and would join one of their tutorial groups in early January 1977. That would allow several months for me to get up to speed and prepare for my second attempt at clerkship.

It came as no surprise when I was assigned a psychiatrist as a new mentor. The administrators were understandably concerned that I might experience another meltdown.

My stethoscope, otoscope, and the personal notebook I'd created were in the dresser drawer—exactly where I'd left them two years earlier. I gathered the book close, like an old friend, and read my notes over and over.

I didn't realize until that moment how much I had missed being a medical student.

The Doctor Is In

CHAPTER TWELVE
CLERKSHIP AGAIN—RAISING LAZARUS

It was awkward joining a class that had been together almost two years. Friendships and patterns of behavior were already well established. There were no large gatherings, so I met my classmates—one tutorial group at a time. They were very welcoming, and I became known as *the golfer*. However, since there was a lot more to me than golf, the label made me feel like I wasn't being taken seriously.

I missed my original classmates who had been scattered to the wind. They were now working as residents in their chosen specialty fields.

Problem-based learning was still at the heart of the tutorial experience. I also enjoyed electives, initially in dermatology, and then later ENT and gynecology. Months flew by, and the dreaded clerkship loomed large in everyone's collective psyche, except for me. I looked forward to revisiting the scene of my personal undoing, and performing well this time.

It was ironic that surgery would be my first clerkship rotation. This time I was assigned a different surgeon—Dr. Joe—a handsome man with an ego to match. The nursing staff swooned in his presence.

There was a rhythm to every day. I'd arrive at the hospital around five in the morning, change into scrubs, grab a coffee in the surgeon's lounge, and meet with my intern and resident. We'd head to the surgical floor, receive a quick report from nursing and the on-call team, and then do rounds with Dr. Joe on his patients. Some of them were new—admitted during the night after assessment in the emergency room. Others were recovering from surgeries performed a few days before. And then we'd head to the operating room for pre-planned elective procedures, and we would work the emergencies into the schedule, too.

The system is hard to describe to a non-medical reader. While there were so many moving parts, they somehow all came together—day after chaotic day. However, there were always unexpected glitches.

For instance, one morning became derailed by the wrong equipment. Let me explain: Dr. Joe had opened the abdomen of an obese middle-aged woman who needed removal of her gallbladder—it was full of stones. I was standing opposite the surgeon, exposing the operative area with a retractor, when Dr. Joe asked the scrub nurse for a particular instrument. He realized instantly it was not his favorite forceps, and it was discovered they were using a tray of instruments prepared for Dr. Bill. You see, every surgeon had his or her preferred tools, and the operating staff was responsible for delivering the correct tray.

Everyone ducked as Dr. Joe threw the interloping forceps against the wall. I was stunned by his sudden change in demeanor. He barked at the staff; a charge nurse was summoned, and a fresh set of instruments was demanded. They had to be autoclaved—cleaned. And somewhere outside the operating room there was a flurry of activity. Dr. Joe fussed and fumed impatiently as the minutes ticked by.

Finally, the door flew open, and a circulating nurse rushed in carrying a silver tray of fresh instruments. Unfortunately, she tripped and fell. Scalpels, forceps, and retractors clanged to the floor, bouncing in all directions. And then Dr. Joe exploded, spewing expletives that would have made a cab driver blush. The patient was stable—much more than the surgeon—and Dr. Joe raced out of the room. Was he coming back?

The charge nurse reassured me that the surgeon would be back, and another set of instruments was prepared. She insinuated that this was not the first time this sort of drama had taken place.

Sure enough, Dr. Joe returned and completed the operation in a calm, professional manner. Not a word of apology was spoken.

This was not his last display of temper. About a week later, I was washing before surgery. This involved a five-minute ritual that included cleaning my fingernails with a plastic pick, scrubbing each finger and hand with a disposable brush, and rinsing from the fingertips toward my elbows. Once finished, I turned the water off, using a knee to close the faucet. I pushed open the operating room door, using my back, and my arms were bent at the elbow while holding them aloft—thus preventing a remaining droplet from running down my forearm and contaminating a hand. Once inside the operating theater, I was greeted by an attendant who helped me don a sterile gown and gloves, without contaminating either of us.

On that particular morning, I made certain to perform every step perfectly because I noticed an infection control nurse—stopwatch in hand—timing every scrub and checking boxes on a form. She was an officious, no-nonsense woman who was afraid of no one, and performed her job with religious zeal.

Then Dr. Joe entered the room. We were about to start a procedure when Ms. Clipboard entered, cleared her throat, and addressed the surgeon. "Dr. Joe, your scrub only lasted two and a half minutes, and I'd like you to step outside and re-scrub appropriately."

Was this woman crazy? No one ever challenged Dr. Joe, and we collectively held our breath. The gauntlet had been dropped.

As expected, Dr. Joe exploded. And then he did something unexpected. He ripped off his gloves and made the first incision bare-handed. Everyone gasped as the infection control nurse wrote furiously. He spoke about how insane scrubbing was anyhow, and how the world had gone mad with all its rules?

At the completion of the hernia repair, there were administrators and several staff surgeons waiting in the hallway. We didn't see Dr. Joe again for a few weeks, and I can only imagine all the emergency committee meetings that were convened.

The patient was watched carefully for any signs of infection. However, he recovered normally, to everyone's relief.

I finished my rotation with a different surgeon. Aside from this drama, I'd become familiar with some of the conditions that required the skill of a general surgeon, such as: an acute abdomen, bowel obstructions, colostomy placements, appendicitis, incarcerated hernias, and abdominal cavities riddled with cancer. My anatomy and pathology books had come to life. I now had a better understanding of how to prepare a patient for surgery and what could go wrong post-op.

Unfortunately, the operating theater would remain a stressful place for me throughout my career. I became an acceptable first assistant, in spite of the fact that my stomach was always in knots. And my near-fainting episodes were predictable if the procedure lasted more than an hour. And yet my patients and their families were thrilled when I was in the room during surgery—they felt safe.

It was a minor miracle that I survived this surgery rotation.

***

Hamilton General Hospital was the scene of the next challenge—two months of immersion on a medical floor, the emergency department and intensive care. This ancient hospital was located in a rough-and-tumble neighborhood and served as the regional trauma center. The first day was devoted to orientation. I was given a beeper and a room key because I was the on-call clerk that night.

I was unable to sleep—not even for one minute. My mind was busy imagining every possible scenario that might occur: a cardiac arrest, acute heart failure, status asthmaticus, a comatose patient, an overdose. It felt like I was cramming for a final exam—endlessly going over memorized facts and protocols—never knowing what the question might be. At least there would be senior people attending to these crises too. Everything did not fall on my shoulders—yet.

Miraculously, I did not receive a single page all night. Of course I called the hospital operator repeatedly to be certain there was nothing wrong with my beeper. In the morning, after shaving and showering, I made my way to the medical floor where I reported to the intern, resident and staff physician. I was assigned four cases. My responsibilities included visiting the patients, documenting their history, and writing daily progress notes. I helped develop the diagnoses and treatment plans, too.

An awkward system called SOAP—Subjective, Objective, Assessment, and Plan—was used for documenting diagnoses in the patient's chart. If done correctly, it was an exercise in tedium and redundant statements. At the same time, the staff physicians did not follow this template. Instead, their notes made liberal use of Egyptian hieroglyphics or Chinese characters—their herky-jerky penmanship was diagnostic of caffeine intoxication. Only the nursing staff seemed capable of making sense of the scribbling.

Every day, I made entries into my personal little black book: protocols, algorithms, mnemonics, and pearls of wisdom on the management of every conceivable patient conundrum. My base of knowledge was expanding almost exponentially.

Several weeks later, an on-call experience still remains fresh in my memory. A routine evening was interrupted by an overhead announcement and the chirping of multiple beepers. There was a cardiac arrest in the Emergency Department. I raced to the scene, and the resuscitation drill was well underway. A resident by the name of Frank—an original classmate of mine—was shouting an order to stand clear. With paddles in hand, he defibrillated the patient into a normal heart rhythm, but not for long.

He turned and ordered me to obtain arterial blood gases—stat. I grabbed the syringe and tried to puncture the radial artery located in the wrist. However, the patient slid back into a pulseless arrest, and I fumbled to obtain a sample. The femoral artery in the groin could not be located either.

Between chest compressions and repeated defibrillations, Dr. Frank yelled, asking if there were any blood gas results. I stammered, "No. I can't find a pulse."

Obviously annoyed, he grabbed the syringe from my hand and angrily plunged the needle into the patient's chest—securing a sample directly from the heart. His gesture took my breath away. The sample would be useless because he wouldn't know whether it was venous or arterial blood.

Dr. Frank was panicked and disorganized—in stark contrast to the obstetrics resident who I had observed manage the emergency Cesarean section several years earlier. It was readily apparent to me that a truly effective clinician had to be more than simply book smart.

The chaos was interrupted by an urgent page. A car accident victim was five minutes away from the trauma center and had no vital signs. Dr. Frank ordered the intern to attend to that case.

While the resuscitation efforts on the Emergency room patient continued, another arrest code sounded. It was a patient on the fifth floor—the medical ward—in a completely different building. Dr. Frank instructed me to go and lead the arrest efforts.

I ran down the dark hallways and up an old, spooky stairwell, as though I was still a member of my high-school track team. While channeling the calm demeanor of the obstetrics resident, I started CPR. A nurse briefed me by reading from the chart. The patient was in ventricular fibrillation. I gripped the paddles for my first time, closed my eyes, and administered the shock—somehow without electrocuting myself or anyone else. It was a miracle! The lethal irregular heartbeat was replaced by a normal sinus rhythm. The patient regained consciousness just as Dr. Frank arrived. He ordered me to leave and assess a patient in another ward who the nursing staff could not arouse.

After another mad dash, I arrived at the bedside to discover a middle-aged male who appeared to be sleeping. His vital signs were stable. A quick reading of the chart indicated that he was a homeless individual who had been found down in a local city park two days earlier. He'd been admitted with a diagnosis of pneumonia and was being treated with antibiotics, bronchodilators, oxygen, and chest physical therapy. This bearded, longhaired gentleman had no teeth and was extremely malnourished. He had been described as being quite talkative but he was quiet now. In fact nothing I did—forcefully rubbing his sternum or pinching his fingernail beds—resulted in even the slightest grimace. He was comatose alright.

I could barely read the notes in my book about the causes of coma—it was in the middle of the night and the lighting was poor. Had the patient experienced a stroke, a seizure, a drug side effect, or was he septic? Maybe he was suffering from some metabolic derangement, like an electrolyte disorder, uremia, or hypoglycemia? He was not a diabetic and was not receiving insulin.

There were no abnormal physical findings, and he was not hypoxic. I had to do something, and so I ordered lab tests: a complete blood count, chemistry panel, and a stat blood sugar.

His blood sugar was reported at eighteen—evidence of severe hypoglycemia—perhaps due to his cachectic state. This sounded preposterous. I'd never heard of a glucose level this low and asked for it to be repeated. Two minutes later the result was shouted out—twenty!

I frantically grabbed my *Washington Manual*, flipped through to the index looking for severe hypoglycemia, speed read the recommended treatment, and ordered a 50-cc syringe preloaded with concentrated glucose. After connecting this massive syringe to the existing intravenous port, I slowly infused its entire contents.

Nothing happened.

As I was disconnecting the syringe, the patient suddenly sat bolt-upright, as though he'd been jet-propelled off the mattress. It scared the living crap out of me and the nurse. We both jumped to attention as the patient turned and said, "What the f*** is going on here?"

One minute he had been corpse-like, the next he was combative and spewing expletives.

Orders were given to continue IV D5W—a sugary intravenous solution—and to make certain that the patient had something to eat. After hastily writing a note, I raced to rejoin Dr. Frank and the intern. I gave them a full report and learned that the only cardiac arrest patient still surviving was the patient I'd defibrillated ninety minutes earlier.

Within the hour, I was summoned back to the homeless man's bedside—he was unresponsive again. I administered another 50-cc bolus of sugar-rich intravenous fluid. This time I was prepared when he abruptly sat up and yelled obscenities again. Someone smarter than me would have to manage this man's hypoglycemia. Mercifully, the sun was coming up, and his attending physician was about to make rounds. I was off the hook for now.

***

My clerkship year continued to unfold. Aside from patient care, I was expected to attend and, at times, present at weekly rounds. This involved choosing a patient whose diagnosis was uncertain; preparing slides of the history taken and the tests ordered; presenting the case to a room full of staff physicians and other learners, and leading a discussion around possible explanations and treatment options. It can't be overstated how valuable this exercise proved to be. Time after time, another attending doctor or the chief resident would offer a new idea, and the patient's problem would be solved.

However, these rounds were quite stressful for all the learners in attendance, especially the intern and clerk who were presenting. There was little time to prepare, and any deficiencies in the work-up or core concepts were quickly exposed. I recall being singled out and grilled by a staff physician that was well known for his derogatory comments. His diatribe was interrupted by a calming voice, "Dr. Campbell. With all due respect, I'm here to learn, and I don't find your sarcastic comments helpful at all. I am not a moron."

You could have heard a pin drop.

I looked around to find out who had spoken, only to discover that the words had come from me! I was more shocked than anyone else in the room. It was the first time I ever recall speaking out in that manner. Usually I found a way to run from a threat. Now I was prepared to fight. The peculiar thing is that I actually developed a warm relationship with this specialist, and would refer to him often in the future. However, I'm getting ahead of myself.

***

The on-call experience every four or five nights

was exhausting. After working the entire day on a ward, I would inevitably be up all night and then have to attend to patients the next day, too. This meant I was routinely awake for forty hours at a time: making important decisions, prescribing drugs, ordering tests, preparing for rounds, and trying not to make a mistake. On looking back, I was clearly impaired during those long hours of sleep deprivation.

You have no idea what I and the other clinical clerks witnessed on a daily basis. There was the homeless person—a well-known alcoholic—who arrived by ambulance, with the right side of his head and mouth caked with coagulated blood. It had been a particularly cold night in the middle of winter, and the patient exhibited obvious signs of frostbite. After methodically removing the blood from his face, it was discovered his ear was missing—it had been torn off. When asked for an explanation, the fellow opened his mouth and spit out the ear! He later explained that his ear had been hurting so much from the cold that he pulled it off and put it in his mouth—to warm it up! You can't make this sort of thing up.

Next, there was the young woman—in an advanced stage of pregnancy—driving at highway speed on a nearby rural highway. She struck a horse standing in the middle of the road—the animal had escaped from its barn. It smashed through the windshield with tremendous force, and the expectant mother sustained multiple injuries. After being extricated from her twisted car, she was transported to the hospital in an unconscious state. The trauma team prepared her for an emergency Cesarean section to save the baby, because a slow fetal heart beat was still detectable. I vividly recall the mother's face. It had been completely pushed in by the impact of the horse's foot—the injury was in the shape of a horseshoe. Of course she died, but her baby survived.

I'll never forget admitting a thirty year old from the nearby Indian reservation. He was about to have yet another reconstructive surgery to repair his face. Several years before, during a depressed and drunken moment in his life, this young man had attempted suicide. He'd placed the barrel of a loaded shotgun under his chin, and, while aiming upward toward his head, pulled the trigger. But he must have jerked, because what he succeeded in doing was blowing his face off—teeth, lips, nose, eyes and eyebrows—all gone. His skull and brain remained intact. Since then, surgically created holes had been fashioned to allow air into the nasal passages. Another stoma served as an opening, through which a straw could be passed, from which he could receive nourishment. Sunglasses were always in place to hide the hideous scars where his eyes used to be. And yet, he exuded happiness and desperately wanted to live.

***

There is no doubt that I could fill this entire book with many other extraordinary cases. But at some point, you would fail to be shocked. And then one example of a human tragedy would blend in with the story before—or the one before that. And that is exactly what started to happen to me.

It was gradual at first. There was a feeling of being detached—a numbness—so that after a while, I couldn't feel anything. I guess it was to be expected. This coping behavior allowed me and other caregivers to function. Otherwise, I'd be constantly crying and incapable of doing anything. However, I did not like it one bit, because my inability to feel soon spread into my personal life. I often felt wooden, like a mannequin, and I laughed a lot less.

True to form, I never mentioned this to my new mentor, the psychiatrist, during our infrequent meetings. He was not Dr. Ron McAuley, and we never really bonded. He always asked many probing questions and remarked about my determination and work ethic since returning to school. I'd explain that there was nothing like driving a cab, failing at competitive golf, being broke, and, at one point, being lost for two years to keep my enthusiasm up.

***

Coming up for air in the spring of 1978, I was greatly relieved that my clerkship was almost over. My evaluations were glowing, and my confidence was at an all-time high. The much feared license exams came and went, and I found them to be intimidating but fair—almost easy—compared with everything else I'd endured. Of course once you know you've passed a test, it's always easy to make a cocky comment like that.

Graduation occurred in late May on a glorious spring day. Dad drove the five hours from Ottawa alone. He thought it best that Mom stay home with Ken, who was studying for high-school graduation exams. However, Dad had an ulterior motive. Aside from being at my graduation, he wanted to see my sister, Sandy. They had been estranged for several years.

My father and Mary Jo were both there on that magical day when I received my hard-won medical degree and recited the Hippocratic Oath. I was a member of the class of 1978, but because of circumstances, I knew very few of them. However, I did become great friends with a classmate, Marianne LeBlanc, and learned about her Bahai faith along the way too.

We hugged and promised to stay in touch.

There was no way to know I'd never see this talented young doctor again because she passed away a few short years later. After all the training and effort involved, her premature death seemed so unfair. It was a painful reminder that "the wolf" was always at the proverbial door.

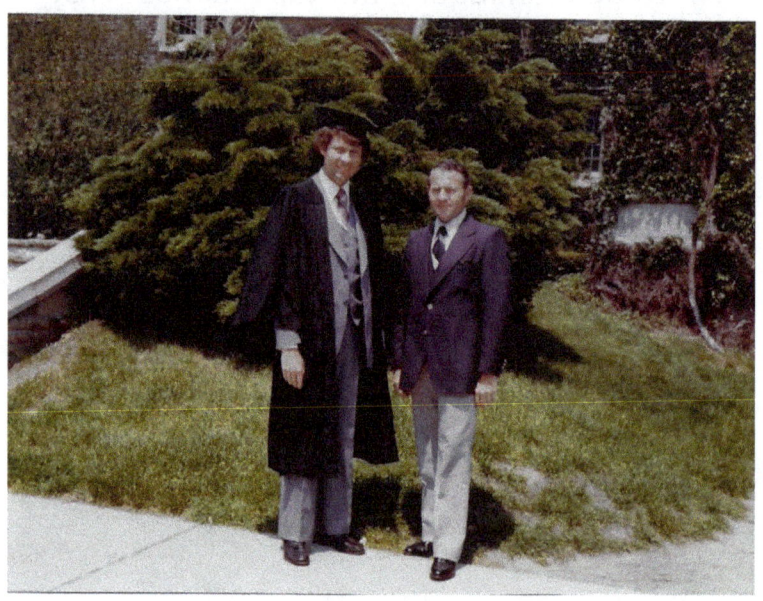

My father and me at my graduation, 1978

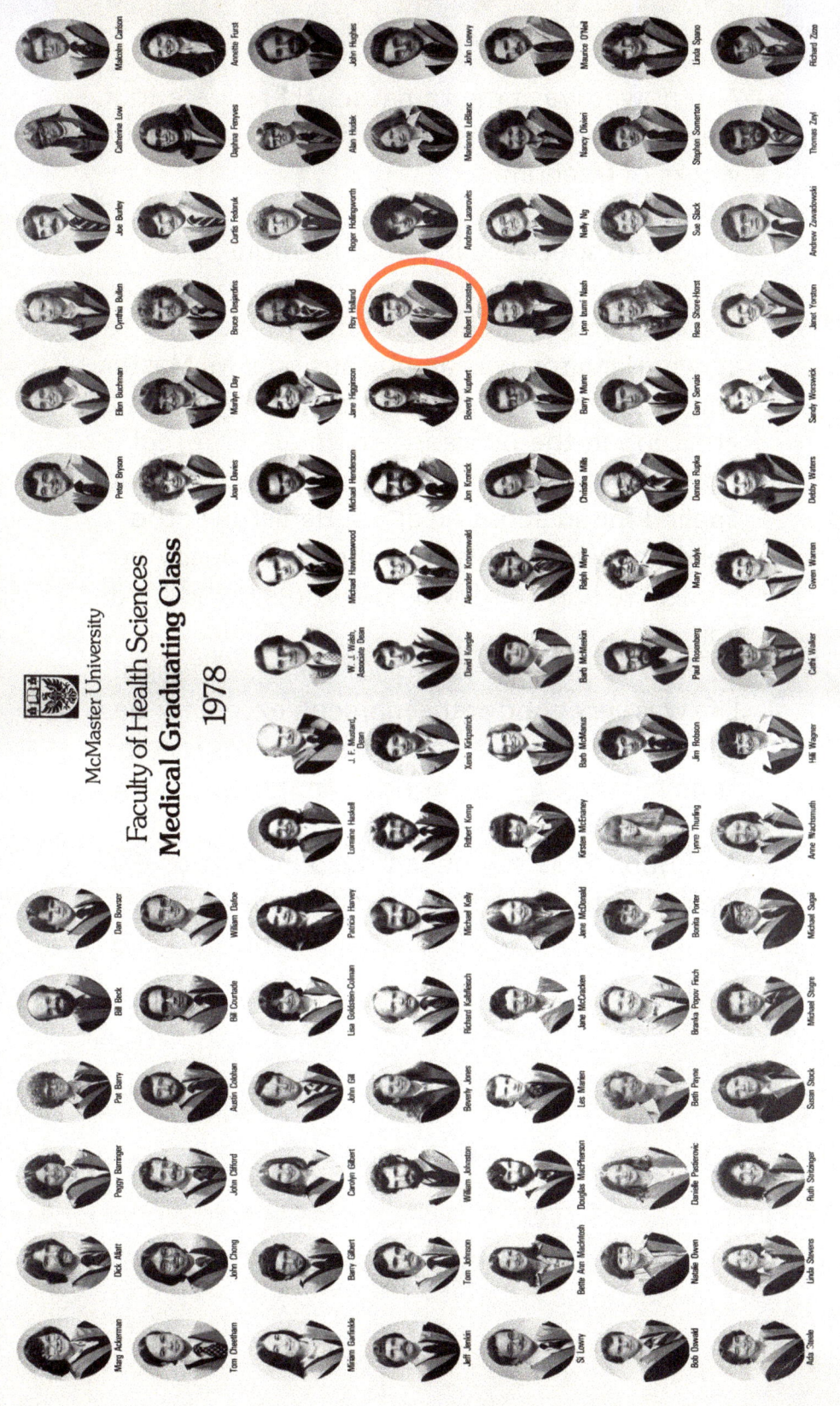

And now it was time to pause. There were four weeks before internship started—four precious weeks of freedom!

I chose to specialize in family medicine and was accepted into the residency programs in London, Toronto, and at McMaster too. The decision to stay in Hamilton was an obvious one: McMaster had a superb residency program, Mary Jo had a great job in the operating room at St. Joseph's Hospital, her family lived nearby, and we had applied for an adoption at the Hamilton Catholic Children's Aid Society. Hamilton was clearly our home. We had put down deep roots in this hard-hat town.

Life was very good at the moment, except for our infertility difficulties which were not responding to any of the treatments popular at the time.

And Bobbi was still buried deep in the closet—hiding her truth from the world's prying eyes.

CHAPTER THIRTEEN
ZEBRAS I HAVE COME TO KNOW

Mary Jo dropped me off at the entrance to McMaster University Medical Center. I caught sight of myself as I approached the front door: long white coat; "Dr. Bob Lancaster" neatly embroidered above my left breast pocket; white shirt and tie; khakis; stethoscope draped around my neck; briefcase in hand; nervous, but ready to make my mark and save the world.

I strode on the multi-colored striped carpet, making sure not to look down. I'd learned as a medical student that if I focused on the patterns of this entrance way rug, they blurred and disoriented me. But it was a difficult flooring surface to avoid because it ran the entire length of the main hallway—a couple of hundred feet.

Turning right, I walked toward the emergency room entrance. Just before that department, there was prominent signage—McMaster Family Practice Teaching Unit—and a glass door on the right. I stopped and paused to read a list of all the doctors who taught in the clinic: Dr. Carl Moore, Dr. John Feightner, Dr. John Evans, Dr. Doug Wilson, and Dr. Vince Rudnick. I had hoped to be assigned to Dr. Moore's practice. He was moviestar handsome, athletic, charismatic, and had a reputation for being a great teacher.

Instead, Dr. Rudnick would be my preceptor. I opened the door, approached the receptionist and was directed into the clinic. Dr. Rudnick's office was the first one on the right, surrounded by three exam rooms. I introduced myself to Shirley Hurst, a nurse practitioner. I'd never even heard of that job title before. Dr. Sol Finkelstein—a resident in his final year—was seated at a desk. He stood, and we were shaking hands when Dr. Rudnick entered the room.

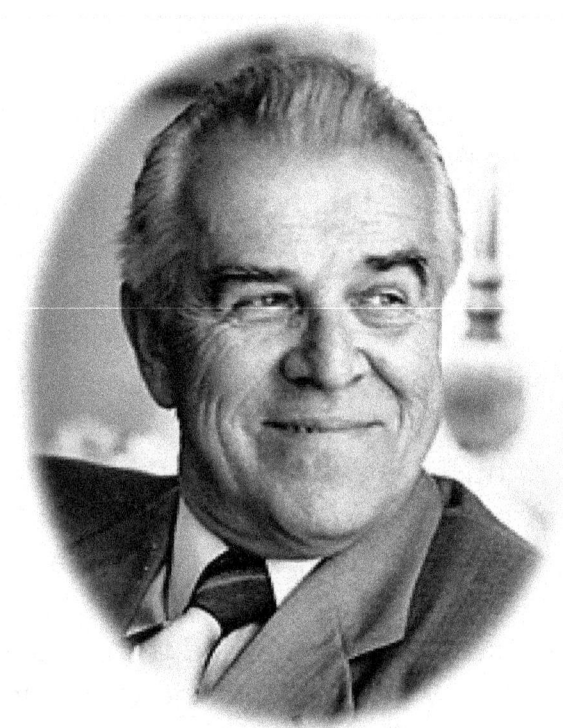

Dr. Vince Rudnick

The Doctor Is In

This beloved Westdale family doctor appeared to be in his fifties: gray hair; stocky; powerful; white shirt and tie; starched white coat. He smelled of Right Guard too. Dr. Rudnick carried himself in a stiff manner and reminded me of my father. In fact, it turned out they were both World War II veterans who loved to spend their free time fishing. Dr. Rudnick was a disciplinarian as well—they could have been brothers.

After a brief orientation, it was time to see patients. About six people were scheduled to see me that first day, and Dr. Rudnick—who liked to be called Vince—watched my every move. Of course I tried to show off and offered multiple diagnostic possibilities for even the simplest of patient complaints. This clearly annoyed him. He spoke in a high voice and reminded me repeatedly that in a family practice, common things are common. "When you hear hoof beats in Hamilton, they are likely being made by a horse and not a zebra."

During the first week, Dr. Rudnick constantly cancelled my orders for tests and labs. He would say, "Treat the patient and the obvious diagnosis. You don't have to confirm everything with a test."

Dr. Rudnick also enjoyed procedures: skin biopsies; sebaceous cyst excisions; drainage of boils; the suturing of lacerations. To be honest, I disliked all of that stuff. Even taking blood and starting intravenous infusions made me squeamish.

Vince and I were not exactly hitting it off, and everything came to a head at the start of my second week. The patient, a twenty-four year old woman named Carole, was new to the practice. She had been encouraged to seek help at our university center because of her mysterious symptoms.

Carole worked for a marketing agency where she delivered lengthy presentations several times a week. About six months earlier, she developed a barely perceptible lisp while addressing her customers. She became self-conscious about her worsening slurred speech and experienced considerable anxiety before each client meeting. There were rumors that she might be drinking or using drugs, and Carole feared that she might lose her job.

She'd seen her family doctor, who told her she was experiencing anxiety and had developed a phobia involving her workplace. Carole was prescribed Valium, which only made her sleepy and did nothing to solve her problem. Meanwhile, her enunciation continued to deteriorate.

After listening to her story and performing a thorough neurological exam, I was convinced I knew the diagnosis. "I'll be right back," I said as I left the room in search of Dr. Rudnick.

He looked like he was about to blow his top when I told him that I thought the patient had myasthenia gravis—a rare neurologic disorder. Dr. Rudnick was red in the face when he gave me his 'common things are common' speech all over again. However, I insisted that my diagnosis was correct. Vince instructed me to sit down and complete my note while he placed a phone call. Shirley bustled into the office because she had heard Dr. Rudnick's voice—it was an octave higher than normal—and she positioned herself between the two of us.

Vince turned to me and said he had Dr. Howard Barrows on the line—the chief of the Neurology Department—and he wanted me to speak with him. I whispered to Dr. Rudnick, "You take the call." I wanted nothing to do with the imposing Dr. Barrows. I'd read his book, heard him speak, and watched him reduce an unprepared intern into a pile of jelly. Vince shoved the phone toward my face.

"Hello, Dr. Barrows. My name is Bob Lancaster, and I'm a brand new intern. I have a young patient in the clinic right now, and I think she has myasthenia gravis. What should I do next?"

I held my breath and waited for his reply. He asked several more questions, ordered me to start an

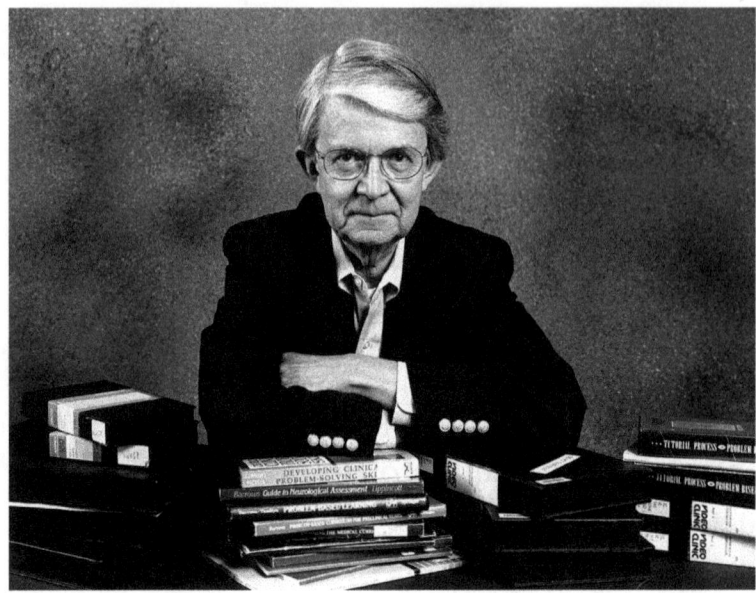

Dr. Howard Barrows

intravenous, and said he'd come down from his office in fifteen minutes.

By some miracle, I successfully placed a butterfly in the patient's right forearm, and Shirley sat with Carole while I paced in the hallway. Dr. Barrows rushed into the clinic waiting room. He appeared right out of central casting: a slender man; unruly grey hair; flowing long white coat; overly large glasses perched precariously on a rather prominent nose; a boyish face—all the while clutching a vial in his left hand. The hospital pharmacist trailed in his wake, like a supporting actor. Apparently, he was curious about the strange test that Dr. Barrows was about to administer.

The Doctor Is In

We entered the examination room where Shirley and the patient were waiting: Dr. Barrows, Dr. Rudnick, the pharmacist, Sol, and me. I emptied the contents of the vial—Tensilon—into a syringe and connected it to the intravenous port. This short-acting drug was capable of almost instantly reversing the signs and symptoms of myasthenia.

Once everyone was seated, I initiated the plan that my patient and I had discussed. She began to read aloud from a magazine I had borrowed from the waiting room. Carole initially enunciated every word perfectly. I urged her to continue at a faster pace and within thirty seconds, her speech began to slur. At the one minute mark, her words became a garbled and dysarthric mess.

I glanced at Dr. Barrows—he nodded—and I injected the drug while holding my breath. Within two seconds, the patient's speech became crystal clear! It was a miracle! Carole stopped reading and sobbed in front of us all.

Everyone exited the room except Shirley. She remained behind to comfort the patient. The pharmacist's eyes were as big as saucers, and Sol looked stunned. Dr. Barrows stared straight at me and said, "Dr. Lancaster, you have just diagnosed the first… and the last case of myasthenia gravis you will ever encounter in your entire career. Congratulations."

With that said, Dr. Barrows bid us all good day and retreated to his office on the top floor. I then referred the patient to his neurology clinic. After a thymectomy and the initiation of maintenance medications, she resumed an almost normal life.

Dr. Rudnick was the last to speak. All he could say was, "I can't believe it," as he shook my hand.

Word of my triumphant diagnosis spread to the other teaching units, and I enjoyed my fifteen minutes of fame. Vince and I resumed our continued tense relationship. He rejected many of my suggestions around new therapies for old conditions, in spite of the fact that I provided references. We appeared to be locked in an unspoken competition that resembled the relationship I had with my father.

Two weeks later, I stumbled upon another diagnosis, and in the process, unintentionally embarrassed Dr. Rudnick. A fifty-eight year old male—David—had been a long-time patient of the practice, and had returned for further assessment of his right wrist pain. He related the following story: It had started six months ago, and there had been no injury. Dr. Rudnick had diagnosed tendonitis and prescribed an anti-inflammatory medication.

The medicine did not help, the pain had now spread up his forearm, and he saw Dr. Rudnick a second time. He was given a steroid injection and told to take it easy. Symptoms persisted and a prescription for physical therapy proved a waste of time. Then Dr. Rudnick referred David to an orthopedic clinic where the diagnosis was confirmed. A cast was applied that ensured the patient rested his arm. Healing was all but guaranteed.

During the four weeks he wore the cast, David experienced no pain. However, as soon as it was removed, the discomfort returned. Now we were face-to-face, and he was obviously frustrated.

I encouraged the patient to tell me about his symptoms. His wrist and now forearm never hurt at rest, and he never was able to find a tender spot. However, when David used his arm repetitively—his hobby was woodworking and involved sawing and other vigorous motions—the discomfort would begin. The first twenty seconds of use were uneventful, but by the one-minute mark, the ache in his wrist and forearm became intolerable. It would force him to stop—the pain would go away—only to recur again after about twenty seconds of reuse. He tried to complete his project, employing many stops and starts until he gave up and returned to Dr. Rudnick.

David's complaint sounded to me like the symptoms of poor circulation—claudication—a condition that occurred in the legs of patients with peripheral vascular disease. But I wasn't sure that claudication could occur in an arm.

I grasped David's hands and was struck by the fact that his right hand was cooler. The pulse in his left wrist was readily palpable. However, I could not locate a pulse in his right wrist or elbow area, and his blood pressure was much lower in this arm too. While listening to his chest, I thought I detected a heart murmur. And the noise became louder over his right collar bone.

David had a major circulatory problem, and his arm was being starved of blood. This time Dr. Rudnick knew better than to lecture me about horses and zebras. He confirmed my findings, and David was referred to a vascular specialist. A large subclavian aneurysm was discovered, and it was loaded with blood clots. After successful surgery, this very grateful patient returned to his woodworking.

Once again, word spread of my diagnostic acumen. While I basked in the limelight, Dr. Rudnick became quieter. He had missed the diagnosis. I felt terrible about the situation. It reminded me of the moment I had diminished my father when I was fifteen years old by beating him at arm wrestling.

Shirley Hurst sensed it was time to intervene.

The Doctor Is In

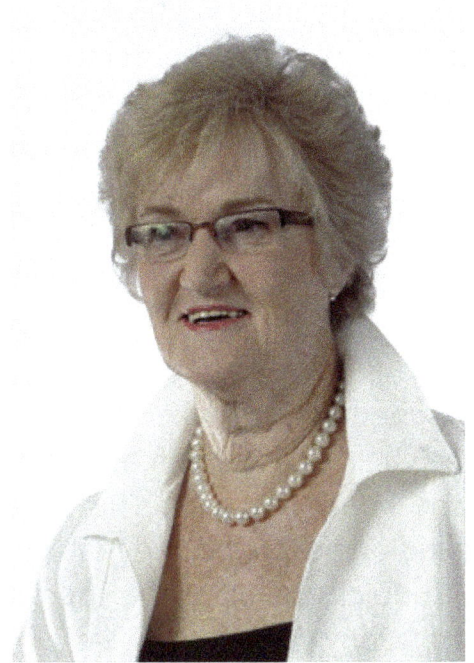

Shirley Hurst

Ms. Hurst was also a beloved figure in the community. She had attended Westdale High School, where she was a star athlete. Shirley went on to graduate from St. Joseph's School of Nursing program, serve in the Canadian Naval Reserve, work in the Emergency Department at St. Joseph's, and eventually receive her Nurse Practitioner degree from McMaster. She went to work for Dr. Rudnick in 1973, and the two of them became a formidable team.

I liked Shirley from my first day in the clinic. She carried herself in a relaxed manner and enjoyed talking about sports between appointments. Her interaction with the patients was something to behold. Shirley listened well, often moving her chair close to signal that the person had her full attention. She also touched an arm or held a hand when appropriate. The patients never felt rushed, and Shirley explained things in terms they could understand. Her bedside manner was something I tried to emulate.

One afternoon, Shirley announced that the two of us were scheduled to make several house calls. I loaded the charts in my briefcase, and she drove because she knew the way. The patients were old and relied on her visits. They talked glowingly about Dr. Rudnick and all of the special care he'd provided for many years.

Shirley suggested that we stop and have a cup of coffee. That's when it became clear she had another agenda in mind. She asked me if I was enjoying my work in the clinic with Dr. Rudnick because, as far as she was concerned, I appeared tense and unsmiling most of the time.

She was right. I wasn't enjoying myself, and it started with what I felt forced to wear. I did not feel comfortable in a shirt, tie and long coat. However, there was an unspoken expectation that I should dress like Vince, or so I thought. Shirley laughed and told me I should arrive for work wearing my version of a professional look.

She recalled the conversation I'd had with her

about my contentious relationship with my father. This made her sad. However, she encouraged me to work things out with my dad and not use Dr. Rudnick as a proxy. Shirley felt that I'd been unnecessarily adversarial and critical of Vince, and my issues were misplaced.

Finally, Shirley provided me with some background information about Dr. Rudnick. She related several examples of his incredible kindness and made me aware of how unusual it was for a physician his age to embrace the new medical school educational model. Shirley reminded me that Vince was one of the few doctors who went out on a limb to hire a nurse practitioner. She finished with the following story: Dr. Rudnick refused to accept McMaster's lucrative offer of employment unless they hired her too. Not only that, he demanded she be made an assistant clinical professor. Apparently there were tense negotiations, and eventually McMaster acquiesced—they needed his large patient base to ensure the success of the teaching unit.

This conversation confirmed that Shirley was one of the wisest, most loyal persons I'd ever met. She gave me a lot to digest. The very next week, I arrived at the clinic wearing one of my nicest golf shirts and a pair of black slacks. Shirley nodded her approval as I hung my white coat behind the door.

It is said that when the student is ready, the teacher will appear. As if on cue, Dr. Rudnick entered the office. It was time for me to learn and listen on a deeper level than I had before. I was prepared to behave in a more respectful manner from that moment forward.

On looking back, I think that marked the day I finally grew up.

CHAPTER FOURTEEN
DR. PAUL O'BYRNE AND ME

In order to specialize in Family Medicine, I needed to complete a two-year residency. During the first year, the candidate was called an intern, and finally, in the second year, a resident. During this training, large blocks of time were devoted to learning in outpatient clinics. Of course, hospital rotations involving pediatrics, obstetrics, gynecology, psychiatry, internal medicine, and emergency care were also mandatory. During every rotation, the trainees returned once a week to the teaching unit they called home. This allowed for the provision of ongoing care for the small group of patients they had developed a relationship with. This was called continuity of care.

My first block of time as an intern with Dr. Rudnick was quickly coming to an end. He would occasionally watch my interaction with a patient behind a one-way mirror. If a complete physical examination was required, I'd offer a gown and leave the room while the patient undressed. Of course, Dr. Rudnick would temporarily close a drape to obscure his view, while the person changed.

One afternoon, a young lady—a beauty pageant winner—was scheduled for her annual health exam and birth control pill renewal. Dr. Rudnick had known Pam and her family since she was a child. Later, I learned that he knew exactly what was about to happen as he positioned himself behind the mirror.

After finishing my history taking, I instructed Pam to change into a gown with the opening to the back. As I was leaving the room, a sudden movement caught my eye. The patient had quickly removed her sundress and was standing in front of the mirror—her magnificent body on full display—as she smoothed her hair. She was totally naked, except for a pair of hoop earrings!

The patient told me there was no need to leave because she was ready for her examination. I became red as a beet, lost my composure, and searched for a comment. Within seconds, Shirley bustled into the room and took control of the situation. She told the patient, in no uncertain terms, to put on the gown. I retreated to the hall where I bumped into Dr. Rudnick. He was wearing a grin from ear to ear.

Apparently this pretty young exhibitionist was known to pull this stunt every year with a new intern. Shirley had been busy with another patient. Otherwise, she would have intervened more quickly. As for Vince—the dirty old man—he was still grinning as Shirley feigned disgust. Times have certainly changed.

A few months later, I was shocked and saddened to learn that Pam had been killed in a car accident. While the details never became public, I often wondered what demons she had been wrestling with.

***

"Hello, Dr. O'Byrne. My name is Bob Lancaster and I'll be one of your interns for the next two months. Do you know where we're meeting this morning?"

"Well hello, Bob. It's wonderful to meet you. My office is over there, just beyond the nurses' station. I'll meet you in five minutes, and please... call me Paul."

Dr. Paul O'Byrne had just arrived from Ireland, and his accent and overall friendly demeanor had caught me off guard. It appeared he would be a benevolent leader.

I joined the two other interns already seated in the tiny office, and we nervously engaged in small talk. After all, we were about to care for a ward full of sick patients, and our every move would be scrutinized by the attending physicians.

Since there were only three of us, we would be on call every third night—an onerous task. After explaining the ground rules and delivering an inspiring pep talk, Dr. O'Byrne assigned ten patients to each one of us. The first day I managed to see every patient and familiarize myself with their diagnoses: pneumonia, congestive heart failure, seizures, fever of unknown origin, hepatitis, cellulitis, delirium, stroke, and ketoacidosis, to name a few.

Every day, discharges and new admissions added to our challenges. However, by the end of the first week, we had all survived an on-call night and had developed a measure of camaraderie. Everything was under control—until it wasn't.

One of the interns became quite ill and would not be able to return to work for weeks. And the other experienced a personal crisis. Her husband was an insulin-dependent diabetic and had literally become blind overnight. She requested a leave of absence—quite understandable given the circumstances—and so I was the last man standing.

Dr. O'Byrne called an emergency meeting. I was panicking because there was no way I could look after the entire ward and be on-call every night. On the other hand, Paul remained cheerful—almost nonchalant—as he pointed out the great opportunity this represented for even more learning. He volunteered to be on call every second night, and we shared the ward duties. There was something special about this budding pulmonologist from Ireland—and saying that we bonded during this rotation is an understatement.

I couldn't help but notice the unusual way in which Dr. O'Byrne recorded his notes in the patients' charts. He did not employ the SOAP method: Instead, he organized his thoughts and diagnoses around bullet points. With the use of arrows, he guided the reader on an investigative and treatment journey. His notes were artistic, resembling a work by Miro—the Spanish painter—who famously explained how he "took a line for a walk" to make his expressive point. Dr. O'Byrne knew how to make his point too.

Of course Dr. O'Byrne did not take credit. He explained that he'd been taught this method by one of his esteemed professors in Dublin. I embraced the technique and have used it throughout my long career. Unfortunately, there aren't any electronic medical record templates that replicate this brilliant charting style.

At the end of the rotation, we shook hands and went our separate ways. Our paths crossed forty years later. Now, Dr. O'Byrne is a world-renowned researcher and the Dean of McMaster Medical School. I'll tell you more about that meeting toward the end of the book.

***

My two years of internship and residency flew by. During this time, I observed just about everything that can go wrong with the human body. The process of going from novice to expert involved enthusiastically embracing every learning opportunity, and putting in countless hours. It required complete immersion and total commitment. There were no shortcuts in the path toward mastery. The acquisition of clinical skills moved along at a dizzying pace.

The old adage of "see one, do one, teach one," perfectly described how I ended up performing procedures I never thought possible—especially for me—the reluctant squeamish one. I can't believe that at one time I performed: circumcisions, lumbar punctures, and bladder taps on septic newborns. I also inserted chest tubes; sutured countless lacerations; drained abdomens full of fluid; injected joints; removed toenails; lanced boils; immobilized broken bones with a cast; and did too many other things to mention.

A long time ago I taught myself how to play golf. It involved closely watching older and more skilled players, and mimicking their technique and course-management decisions. Other lesser players taught me the folly of arrogance, a disorganized regimen of practice and a poorly controlled temper.

This was exactly how I learned the art of being an effective physician. I imitated others until my own unique style and approach emerged. Perhaps it wouldn't work for everyone, but it worked for me.

While I'm on the subject of style, I was fortunate to assist many surgeons. I observed how differently they held a scalpel and performed an incision. Some approached the operative area almost reverently, and made delicate and very precise strokes with the knife—like a Dutch Master painter. Others rushed in, using bold movements that frightened me to death.

One obstetrician in particular employed his usual thrust-and-parry approach when performing a Cesarean section. One time, as he cut through the uterus and the amniotic membrane, he lacerated the baby's cheek below the right eye. The one-inch cut was expertly repaired, but the child would bear the evidence of this surgeon's aggressive technique for the rest of its life.

While assisting this same surgeon on another occasion, I witnessed the successful delivery of another newborn by C-section. However, there was considerable bleeding, and the doctor attempted to place a suture around the offending arterial bleeder. Without a clear view, he dramatically thrust the needle driver into the puddle of blood and secured the ligature. The bleeding stopped, and the rest of the repair was completed uneventfully.

Except several post-partum days later, the new mother developed a fever and severe left flank pain. As it turned out, the suture that had ligated the bleeding artery had also tied off her left ureter. Her recovery now required urology, intravenous antibiotics, and another operation to relieve her left kidney—it had swollen like a balloon from backed-up urine.

I made a mental note that, in the future, I'd only refer to surgeons who possessed a good bedside manner and a painterly touch.

***

Before closing this chapter on my residency training, several more events occurred that have had a lasting impact on me.

First, I was elected to serve as Chief Resident by my peers. The position involved a little more work. However, it was an honor I readily and humbly accepted. I tried to emulate the leadership style of Dr. O'Byrne, and of course I fell short. There is an engraved silver cup memorializing my tenure, which resides in a prominent place in my living room. It was presented to me at our graduation party, as a gesture of thanks, by the family-practice interns and residents.

The Doctor Is In

Second, I received a life-changing phone call during another internal medicine rotation—this time at Hamilton General Hospital. The head nurse located me in a patient's room and told me my wife was on the phone. Mary Jo was still employed in the operating room at St. Joseph's, and it was unusual for her to call me at work. Was she sick? Were her parents alright? Something was wrong. My mind raced as I walked briskly to the phone at the nurses' station. I stretched the cord as far as it would go and lowered my voice.

"Jo, are you alright?" I could barely hear her because there was screaming in the background. "Jo… Jo… what's going on?"

"We have a baby girl! Children's Aid just called! It's a girl! She was born on September 1, 1979—a couple of weeks ago. I'm going home right now."

Mary Jo began to cry and ended the phone call. I became aware of cheers in the background. The well-wishes were coming from the nurses who had gathered around me during my so-called private conversation. They'd heard every word!

I finished my charting, and the staff pushed me out the door. After embracing at home, Jo and I hurriedly prepared for the new addition to our family. We made a dash to the local department store for diapers, baby bottles, formula, clothes, blankets and some toys. A homemade crib had sat idle for years, and now it was time to dust it off. We installed a mobile above the cradle to amuse our new bundle of joy.

The next day, we left the adoption center with Jacqueline Jennifer in our arms. After a quick stop at St. Charles Catholic Church, we introduced her to Mary Jo's parents—their first grandchild—and then returned home to call my parents in Ottawa. For a couple of days, patients, rounds and on-call nights were the farthest thing from my mind.

Jo remained at home with the baby while I returned to my training. And before you knew it, Mary Jo was pregnant, again. However, this time she did not miscarry, and her due date was at the end of August, 1980.

There was no time to waste. I had to finish my residency, find a job, purchase a larger home for a family of four, learn how to be a father, and support Mary Jo through a difficult pregnancy—she had developed toxemia. Her parents helped with the down payment on a home that only a doctor could afford. Not only that, the interest on the mortgage was sixteen percent, and my future was still completely uncertain. If ever there was a time that I might be tempted to crack, this was it.

Instead, I happily soldiered on because this situation was far easier than the hopelessness I faced behind the wheel of a cab just five short years before.

During my last few weeks in the teaching unit, I didn't think there was much Shirley and Dr. Rudnick could teach me anymore. I had seen and done so much, I felt I could handle any conceivable patient problem. However, they were about to deliver one of their most important lessons that showed me I still had a lot to learn.

Mrs. Woods was one of Vince's original patients, and I'd met her on multiple occasions. She had developed advanced cancer and was now too weak to come to the office. I was assigned to visit her at home, and these encounters had become progressively more difficult—especially for me. She had exhausted all the known chemotherapy regimens; thoughts of a cure had long ago been abandoned, and she was fading away.

There was not another test I could offer, and I had no more treatment tricks in my doctor bag. I felt useless to her—impotent—empty of any new suggestions that might save her life. I didn't want to visit anymore because I thought I was wasting her time.

Dr. Rudnick and Shirley became aware of the situation, sat me down, and closed the office door. They alternated speaking and did not mince words as they made their case.

"No matter how smart you think you might be, a point is always reached in the life of every patient where death is inevitable. This is a fact of life. A moment occurs when everything looks hopeless, and there is apparently nothing more to do. In time you'll recognize these inflection points and realize you still have an important role to play: answering questions, allaying fears, supporting family members, guiding them through discussions around advanced directives, and promising to be available until the very end. It's called palliative care. Be prepared, because you'll need to be innovative and think outside the box. It will be a busy time as you treat unwelcome symptoms and ensure that their death is as special as their birth once was, many years ago.

"The patients will enjoy your visits. They will tell you about their lives and more than a few secrets too, because they'll have turned off their filters. You'll learn that being part of a person's inner circle at the time of their passing is a special honor—a privilege."

I'd heard enough and thanked them profusely until they ordered me to stop. It was an important final lesson.

The rigorous board certification exam came and went, and I was relieved to learn that I was a successful candidate. The official start of my career as a family physician was only one month away. My accomplishments up to that point had taken the support of Mary Jo, my family, hard work, luck, Dr. McAuley, Dr. Paul O'Byrne, Shirley Hurst, Dr. Vince Rudnick, and hundreds of supporting cast members.

My wife was ill, a mortgage payment was due, the grass needed cutting, my daughter needed attention, we had a new family car, my residency stipend had come to an end, Bobbi was still in the closet, and I didn't have one patient to call my own.

Some might say the doctor was in trouble—but they would have been wrong. The truth of the matter was: This doctor was in.

The Doctor Is In

CHAPTER FIFTEEN
BREAKING UP IS HARD TO DO

"Hello, Mrs. Robinson. My name is Dr. Lancaster, and I'm Dr. Shea's new partner. Congratulations on the birth of your new baby boy."

"Thank you. Is Dr. Shea here? Will he have time to see me today?"

"No, he's away on a well-deserved vacation. I see you're scheduled for a post-partum check. Are you having any difficulties?"

"Everything is going well (breath). My pregnancy was normal (breath) and the baby came out head first (breath) on my due date (breath). My lactation consultant (breath) has been a big help (breath) and breast feeding is a breeze (breath)."

The baby was perfect in every way. However, I had to ask the obvious question. "Mrs. Robinson—you seem to be quite short of breath, and I've noticed your legs are swollen. Is this a new issue or have you been experiencing these symptoms for a long time?"

The patient said she had noticed increasing shortness of breath for the past week. She blamed it on being out of shape and on the weight she'd gained during the pregnancy. There had not been excessive bleeding at the time of delivery. No one had mentioned anemia in the hospital, and she did not have a history of asthma. However, when I palpated both calves, she winced, and my thumbs left deep indentations in her shins.

I sensed that one of those zebras—the one that made a habit of following me around—was now galloping by the door.

Using my calmest voice, I told the patient that her heart rate and breathing were both faster than expected and that I'd like to order tests. Within the hour I learned she was not anemic. However, the major veins in both legs were loaded with blood clots—the dreaded deep vein thrombosis. Worse yet, I feared some of those clots had already travelled to her heart and were threatening her life.

I directed the patient to the emergency department, where further tests revealed her heart and lungs were clogged with multiple pulmonary emboli. She was admitted to the intensive care unit where she received oxygen, anticoagulants, and various other procedures.

Mrs. Robinson was back in the office a month later to see Dr. Shea for her baby's first immunizations. She regaled him with a colorful account of her recent hospitalization and my involvement. I don't think she fully realized how lucky she was to have survived unscathed.

***

Dr. Phil Shea and I had crossed paths earlier during my training. The residents considered him to be really smart and somewhat demanding—perhaps abrupt is a better word. He was one of the most popular family physicians in the region, and we developed a friendship of sorts. Dr. Shea championed women's health issues, natural childbirth, and the importance of breastfeeding. His waiting room looked more like a combination of an obstetrician and a pediatrician's office. There was literature everywhere about Lamaze classes and the La Leche League. He was also an outspoken, pro-life advocate and a devout Catholic.

There was a lot to like here, including his wife and their many rambunctious children. Their home in the country was noisy, rambling, comfortable and welcoming. It was so different than the neat and orderly manner in which I lived—a result of my obvious obsessive-compulsive tendencies.

Phil wore a full beard when they weren't in style, and his hair was often cropped unfashionably short. He had a perpetually stuffy nose, and resembled a big kid who needed his adenoids removed. He was not preoccupied with his wardrobe and carried himself in an unaffected manner.

Dr. Shea also worked extensively with midwives and participated in many home births. This placed him at odds with the mainstream medical community, and there were more than a few confrontations. Dr. Shea was an individualist, and his maverick tendencies really appealed to me. I chose to join him in practice as his junior partner. We shared an office on the second floor of a nondescript strip mall at Upper James and Mohawk Road.

***

Since I had no practice base of my own, I spent my first few months providing vacation relief for Dr. Shea. I also worked as a *locum tenens* for several other doctors who needed a break.

One of these practices belonged to a well-known downtown family physician. I arrived the first day and glanced at the schedule. There were three patients booked every fifteen minutes, which added up to thirty-six encounters before lunch. Obviously, I didn't know any of the staff or their systems. By noon, I was two dozen patients behind. Everyone was grumbling in the crowded waiting room, and the scheduler was busy dismantling the appointment sheet for the next two weeks—she realized very quickly that I was

The Doctor Is In

incapable of processing patients that quickly.

I did my best. The returning doctor teased me about my lack of productivity, and bragged about his roster size and his Mercedes. I quietly promised myself I would never allow my practice to function like a cash-generating production line. It was the first and last time I walked through the door of that medical factory.

Another practice I covered was located just down the street from our office, and the family physician—Dr. Gibson—alerted me that he had several pregnant patients who were due during his vacation. A woman I'd never met went into labor in the wee hours one night, and she would be my first delivery as a community doctor.

Even though I had quite confidently delivered many babies as a resident, there was always the security of knowing a chief resident or staff physician was right around the corner. Now *I* was the attending physician—alone—at three in the morning. I didn't feel so confident anymore and would have enjoyed someone holding my hand as I applied a vacuum extractor.

The realization that I was now the decider—and totally responsible for a patient's well-being—discomforted me. My bravado rapidly disappeared. I still had a lot to learn about being decisive and taking ownership of my actions.

Several days later, I directed another patient from Dr. Gibson's practice to labor and delivery—her water had broken. An hour later, I received a call from the obstetrical nurse that I'll never forget.

"Your patient is here, Dr. Lancaster. She's in active labor, and we can't find a fetal heart beat!"

"Would you repeat that?"

"There is no heartbeat, and the mother reports not feeling any movement since yesterday. The intern has confirmed our findings too. The baby has died. The patient and her husband are distraught, and I hope you can come quickly. This is her first pregnancy."

Oh my goodness! I'd never experienced a stillbirth during my training, and at that moment, I wished I was a million miles away. Before I left for the hospital, I quickly read about the causes, management, and complications. At least I'd be a few pages ahead of them.

By the time I arrived, the mother was almost fully dilated. I'd never met the couple before, and they were struggling with the unimaginable. There was no time for tears now—she was overwhelmed with the pain of childbirth—and I brought the best of me to the bedside. We locked eyes, and she followed my every command.

The ordeal was intense and mercifully brief. The male infant was perfectly formed; he possessed a striking amount of jet-black hair, the cord and placenta were unremarkable, and the baby's macerated skin was sloughing onto my gloved fingers. A pediatric resident from the nursery obtained cord blood samples and cultures in the hope a cause could be found.

At first, the couple did not want to see the child. After telling them how sad I was for the two of them, I explained the importance of seeing their son.

"Of course it will be difficult," I said. "However, you will regret for the rest of your life not touching him and having a photo. I'd suggest that we provide you with a lock of his hair too. You've got to trust me on this one."

They held their boy. He was swaddled in a blue blanket—his cute little face was all that was visible. I asked if they were Catholic, and they nodded their heads. I offered to baptize the baby, and the request caught them off guard. They readily consented and looked on as I poured water on the tiny forehead and recited those magic words: "I baptize thee, in the name of the Father, the Son, and the Holy Spirit. Amen."

At the time, I was still a devout Catholic. It was later that I fell away from organized religion, when the Church turned its back on me, and other transgender individuals like me.

My textbook indicated that there was often a great deal of guilt experienced by the mothers of stillborn children. And the divorce rate was much higher too!

I wonder what ever happened to that couple. They were both in their late thirties, and another pregnancy would have been a high-risk undertaking.

Not that I had any say in the matter, but stillbirth was one more thing on my growing list of medical diagnoses that I hoped I'd never have to experience again—professionally or personally.

***

My first summer in practice flew by. Around the middle of August, Mary Jo was hospitalized for toxemia. Her mother cared for Jennifer during the week, and I could hardly wait to be with my little girl on the weekends. Meanwhile, I was covering for Dr. Shea's deliveries, too—he had signed out to me because he was enjoying a rare bit of freedom that a new partner afforded.

Sure enough, one of his patients went into labor on a Saturday morning, and little Jenny and I were off to St. Joseph's. The obstetrical nurses cared for her while I delivered the new baby. Jenny was eleven months old, and wasn't walking yet. She still had a heart-shaped vascular nevus—a birthmark—clearly visible on her forehead, and the red splotch made her even more precious.

It wasn't the last time I brought Jenny to labor and delivery when I should have been home.

Two weeks later, it was our turn. The obstetrician induced labor in Mary Jo, and she failed to progress. Finally, Laura Alexis was born on August 29, 1980, by C-section. Laura was in great shape, but Jo experienced rigors and fevers post-op. She was septic. Of course I feared she would die, and I had no idea how I would cope with a new baby, a one-year-old, and my professional life. I was barely holding on as it was.

Thankfully, Mary Jo recovered and was discharged home. Now I was even more available to grow my practice. I'd become disenchanted with providing relief for vacationing doctors and accepted a position as an attending physician at an inpatient facility—Chedoke Continuing Care Center—the four C's. The old building was once a sanitarium where patients recovered from tuberculosis. Now it served as home to individuals who required long-term care for advanced multiple sclerosis, severe cerebral palsy, Huntington's chorea, Friedreich's ataxia, traumatic brain injury, severe strokes, and spinal cord catastrophes. The only family that many of these patients knew was the staff. It was an honor to minister to this group of patients, and my real world learning continued at a rapid pace.

***

Meanwhile, back at the office, people were clamoring to roster with me: nurses; speech, occupational, and physical therapists; some golf buddies; Hamilton Streets and Sanitation employees I had worked with; cab driver acquaintances; professors; high school teachers; nuns; Catholic priests; neighbors and friends. My practice was growing exponentially, and it was a heady and humbling experience. The pressure was on to perform.

First, I would evaluate every new patient and establish a game plan that sometimes required a lab test or a specialist referral. Then, I would ask the office workers—Dr. Shea's original staff—to process my requests. Later, I would find out they spoke with him, and Dr. Shea frequently decided my investigations were unnecessary. They cancelled my orders without me knowing.

He was likely unaware of the impact of his actions, but this was the start of the unraveling of our relationship.

During this time, I was perfecting my approach:

learning how to cajole frightened children with dolls and distraction; refining my explanations and analogies; discovering what things motivated my patients to change unhelpful habits; learning how to administer shots that a patient wouldn't feel; developing a roster of trusted specialists, and creating an efficient pattern to my work day.

There were so many moving parts: assessing twenty or more office patients a day; attending to the sickest ones in the hospital; assisting at surgeries; completing charts in the medical record department; performing house calls; meeting patients at the fracture room where I'd apply casts to stabilize broken bones; visiting nursing homes; making time for the Four C's facility; attending educational rounds, and teaching.

Yes, I was asked to teach medical and nursing school students at McMaster. I was given a title—Assistant Clinical Professor—and routinely had a learner in the office. Sometimes it was hard for me to believe that I had been one of those students just a few years before—fumbling to try to take a blood pressure.

It was also expected that I participate on hospital committees. I also volunteered in the community and particularly enjoyed being on the Board of Directors of Catholic Children's Aid—the organization where we had adopted Jennifer. In fact, during a tumultuous time in its history,

I served as President of the Board.

During my tenure, I became aware of an older child who was in need of a loving family. His name was Timmy, born in January of 1983, and he had been placed for adoption by his Cree Indian mother shortly after birth. Timmy had fetal alcohol syndrome and was busy fighting for life. He'd survived open-heart surgery, numerous pulmonary infections, and now he was being bounced from one foster home to the next.

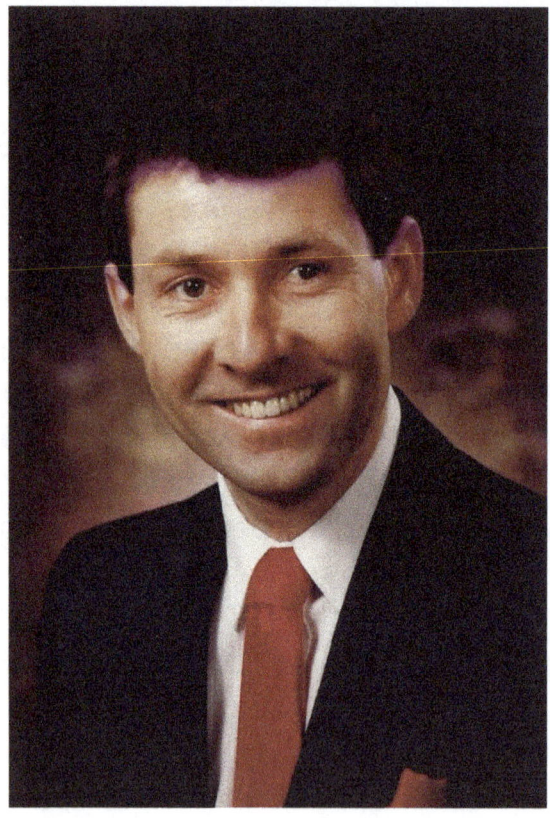

Dr. Bob Lancaster, circa 1982

Timmy couldn't swallow; he was tube fed, and had not uttered a word yet—even though he was well over a year old—when I stumbled upon his story.

Something about his cute little face that had accompanied an advertisement in the paper called out to me. I voiced my concern and interest to Mary Jo, who was busy at home with our two girls. At the time, they were three and four years of age.

Together we visited Timmy in Toronto—he was hospitalized at the time—and fell in love. We changed his name to Jeffery Robert, completed the adoption papers, and brought him home. This was during the spring of 1984, and was just in time for my fifty-seven year old father to get to know him.

Dad died suddenly and unexpectedly later that year, in August. He had a heart attack—in his sleep—after spending the day with me building a swing-set for his grandkids. After he died, I remember feeling numb and forcing myself not to cry. There was no way that I could break down because there were too many balls in the air. In every direction I turned, someone was depending on me.

***

During my first couple of years in practice, not many of my new patients had become pregnant yet, and I wanted to keep my obstetrical skills intact. So I asked if I could tag along on some of Dr. Shea's deliveries. He agreed, and I found myself at a home-birth with Phil and a young couple that I would best describe as free spirits.

The couple lived in a sparsely furnished rental along with a few pets. My job was to hold a gigantic dresser mirror at the foot of the bed so the mother could gauge her progress with every push. The setting was an old mattress that had lost its springiness. The weight of her pelvis created a crevasse into which all the instruments gravitated. The crowning head of the newborn was barely visible deep in the recesses of the ancient Sealy Posturepedic.

Dr. Shea remained unruffled.

And then there was a baby's cry. A dozen cats and dogs descended on the source of the noise— vigorously licking the baby. As if this wasn't enough, the new mother and her attendants requested the placenta, which they grilled and served later in the day—as a celebratory meal. I felt like I had entered the twilight zone.

And Dr. Shea continued to remain unruffled.

I was trying to keep an open mind about home

births, but this experience left me with more questions than answers.

***

Of course, not everything revolved around obstetrics. For example, I received a call from Dusty—a street sweeper who worked for the City. He was concerned about a co-worker, George, who had become ill and was unable to get out of bed. I'd met both of them when I worked for Streets and Sanitation, twelve years earlier. They remembered I was going to be a doctor and had seen a recent notice in the paper.

Dusty reminded me that he had watched, along with all the other laborers, as I received my first driving lesson from the foreman. The memory of the incident caused both of us to laugh. You see, I was eighteen at the time—madly in love—and had arranged to pick up my date in a borrowed car. Except I didn't have a license and had never driven a vehicle—not counting my bicycle and a peddle car I got for Christmas when I was six.

So, I'd pestered the foreman—Ollie Wilson—to teach me how to drive, and, after several days of begging, he threw me the keys to the water truck. We were on our lunch break, and the entire crew exited the lunch room and watched as I climbed into the cab. The tank was half full with water—two thousand gallons—and to make matters worse, the truck had a clutch.

"Don't hit anything," Ollie yelled, as I depressed the clutch and started the engine. I was barely underway when it stalled. And I stalled the vehicle repeatedly. Finally, I aggressively revved the engine and engaged the clutch. This time, the truck lurched forward violently, and then stalled again. Except now, the water sloshed toward the cab with great force, propelling the vehicle several feet off the ground. It landed with a bang. Now the water raced backward and slammed into the rear of the tank, and the truck jumped backwards two feet. This cycle repeated over and over. I felt like I was atop a bucking bronco, and the workers—Dusty included—were clutching their sides as they laughed uncontrollably and fell from their cheap seats.

And now Dusty wanted me to help a very sick friend. A house call was required. I knocked on the door of a sparsely appointed apartment, was guided to the bedroom, and immediately realized that George was in serious condition.

He had been working two weeks earlier when he developed nausea and profound weakness—he'd been losing weight too. I reintroduced myself and noticed George was jaundiced. His liver was enlarged and hard—as though it had been replaced with a bag of rocks. He was in considerable pain.

The Doctor Is In

It was impossible to sugarcoat the diagnosis, and George demanded the truth from me. It was cancer—likely spread from his bowel or pancreas—and he did not have a lot of time left. George declined transfer to the hospital, agreed to take pain medicine, and thanked me for telling it like it was.

I arranged home care and promised to visit again in two days. Dusty was relieved to finally know what was wrong with his buddy.

Two days later, George passed away!

I read the obituary in the paper and wasn't sure if it was appropriate for a doctor to visit the funeral home of a patient. I took a chance and was warmly greeted by Dusty and a dozen other city workers. And then I was introduced to George's girlfriend—Lacey—and offered my condolences.

All hell broke loose. In front of a hundred people, she accused me of killing her boyfriend with my pain pills. "He had been doing alright until you arrived!" She couldn't believe that I had the nerve to show up at his visitation. "You should be ashamed of yourself."

Red-faced and mortified, I slithered out the side door of the funeral home and vowed I would never again get involved with a grieving family I didn't know.

It had become apparent to me that the actual practice of medicine sometimes involves tip-toeing through a field of emotionally charged landmines. I had not been prepared for this challenge.

***

I remember the day when shock waves spread through the primary care community. A young family physician—just like me—had been busily growing his practice when the unthinkable happened. He had been treating an asthmatic thirty-eight year old male when he discovered his patient had hypertension. Apparently, the man had a long family history of blood pressure elevation that had contributed to strokes, renal failure, and heart attacks. Obviously, it was important the patient receive treatment to normalize his pressures.

Unfortunately, the physician prescribed a beta-blocker. This class of drugs was often used to treat hypertension. However, it can also cause bronchospasm and should not be used by an asthmatic.

Why was the doctor unaware of this history? Perhaps the pharmacist did not know the patient was using inhalers to control his wheezing. Maybe the handout that accompanied the medicine was ignored.

In any event, the patient swallowed the medicine and experienced an ever-increasing shortness of breath. His puffers were ineffective, panic ensued, a respiratory arrest followed, and the young man passed away.

A coroner was involved, as well as lawyers, licensing organizations, and reporters. The doctor's name and all the unpleasant details—including heart-wrenching comments from the family of the deceased—became compulsory reading in the local newspaper, and the topic of conversation among my colleagues. His reputation was shredded.

We physicians agreed that a blunder this obvious should never have happened.

However, we collectively crossed our fingers and hoped that nothing like this would ever happen to us. But, as we knew, the list of things that could go wrong was a long one and included: a prescribing error; a missed, wrong, or delayed diagnosis; an abnormal lab test that went unnoticed; a charting deficiency; the failure to inform a patient; an overlooked screening test—just to name a few. The importance of an organized practice with fail-proof systems and a conscientious staff were mandatory. However, there was always the human factor and something capricious called *luck*.

On one hand, I attempted to use best-practice recommendations that were in keeping with other family doctors in the community. This included staying up to date and practicing within the scope of my specialty. And when I didn't know something, I did not allow my ego to get in the way—ignorantly plowing forward and potentially harming a patient.

On the other hand, I was also engaged in home births—a high-risk activity that drew condemnation from almost every obstetrician, pediatrician, and family physician in the community. Except for Dr. Shea and a few midwives, delivery at home was considered a high-stakes gamble. Of course we scoured the medical literature for studies and papers that supported our activities. There were just enough to keep us emboldened.

Once I attended my first delivery at home, the word was out, and I became the darling of the midwifery community. And there was definitely a very small group of consumers who appreciated the service. They were an eclectic bunch: free spirits; chiropractors; members of the Church of Scientology; and several farm families—to name a few. They shared a similar sentiment: intense dislike of mainstream medicine and all the attendant intervention that went along with it.

Most of my deliveries took place in a hospital

setting where contemporary birthing centers had been created to simulate a home. However, even this accommodation failed to entice the home birth crowd.

I made every attempt to be certain a planned birth at home involved a truly low-risk pregnancy. And I carried oxygen and a black bag full of equipment too.

During the writing of this memoir, I reviewed a little green book in which I had recorded every birth I ever attended. I was surprised that the total exceeded one thousand. Of that total, only eighteen planned home births ever took place under my care. I'm happy to report that there were never any problems.

However, on two occasions, midwives called me to the homes of their private patients—where labor was not progressing. Transfer to hospital had became mandatory. These midwives were pleased that I was the one explaining their case to a hostile on-call obstetrician, who reprimanded me for being involved in home deliveries.

While I'm on the topic of obstetrics, I'll never forget delivering the wife of one of my golf buddies in the hospital. Her pregnancy was entirely unremarkable, as was the delivery. In fact, there was no evidence of even a tiny vaginal tear. A few minutes after delivery of the placenta, she and her husband were admiring their new baby boy when I heard what sounded like running water.

I lifted the bed sheet and was surprised to see a large and growing puddle between her legs. Blood was pouring out from her vagina, like a wide open spigot. There was not a second to waste. The baby was whisked away; I massaged the uterus and evacuated a large clot; syntocinon was administered; an intravenous started; blood was ordered, and an obstetrician was called. Still, the bleeding continued.

My golf friend looked up at me and asked, "Is everything alright?"

I lied and said everything was fine, and that we saw this amount of bleeding sometimes. At right about that moment, his wife—now white as a sheet—lost consciousness. The head of the bed was lowered, more syntocinon administered, intravenous normal saline was infused full bore, and I forcefully squeezed her uterus between my two hands—one inside her vagina and the other on her lower abdomen.

The transfusion commenced at just about the same time the patient awoke and the obstetrician strode into the room. Everything was now under control. This was the closest I ever came to losing a mother. It was situations like this that had filled old graveyards I'd noodled around when I was younger. There were frequent markers from the 1800s, indicating the burial place of a young mother and an infant child.

There is no doubt in my mind that if this complication had taken place during a home birth, the patient would have died, and my story would have been on the front page of the newspaper at the time of the inquest.

After this episode, I decided not to participate in home births anymore. However, several patients that I'd delivered before at home had a way of twisting my arm.

***

"Marilyn, I'm not going to refill your narcotic prescription from another doctor."

"Dr. Lancaster, my doctor is away, and I'm running out of pills. I was told you were kind. You're turning out to be mean, and I'm not going to leave until you renew my prescription."

Marilyn was a parishioner at St Charles Church, the very place where Mary Jo and I were married. We also had our children baptized there and regularly attended services. My father-in-law was an architect and had designed this unusual facility. It was semi-circular in shape, which allowed the priest to face the entire congregation while saying Mass—the original theater in-the-half-round.

I had often seen a strange looking woman—Marilyn—attending Mass. She was in her sixties; cachectic; bleached blond hair; pancake makeup, and often dressed in a negligee—in church!

Apparently, she approached the pastor, Father Sherlock, and requested that he find her a new doctor. Now I was face to face with this peculiar woman, and things were not going well. I explained that she did not have a condition that warranted narcotic use. If she were to become a patient, I would insist we gradually taper and stop this medicine and explore other treatment regimens.

Marilyn was not listening, and her demands for narcotics became louder. She threatened that if I didn't give her the prescription, she would kill herself. I remained firm in my recommendation, and she noisily left the office—slamming every door in her path.

A minute later, a patient ran into the office—breathless—as he described witnessing a woman intentionally dive head first down the stairwell a few seconds earlier. I raced to the lower landing and discovered Marilyn in a heap—unconscious and bleeding profusely from her nose and ears.

Paramedics were called, and she was transported to the trauma center. Many months passed, and she was back at church. Marilyn now appeared to be cognitively impaired, and her speech was slurred. She could barely open her mouth as she spoke because of the fractured jaw she had sustained. Perhaps it was still wired shut. Her entire story was tragic.

There was never a dull moment in the life of a busy family physician.

***

I'm embarrassed to share with you that I have never dealt with conflict very well. I learned to be silent—and not be punched—when my father went off on one of his many alcohol-fueled rages. Demanding authority figures frightened me.

Initially, Dr. Rudnick intimidated me with his militaristic style and rigid pronouncements.

Dr. Phil Shea was a dominant fellow, too, and I cowed and followed his lead around pro-life issues and home births. Shirley Hurst was not around to help guide me through this mess.

Phil gave me the impression that he didn't appreciate my diagnostic acumen. His staff remained devoted to him, even though I was paying half their salary. I attended pro-life rallies in an effort to understand what Dr. Shea was so passionate about. One gathering was led by another family doctor who spewed dogma and hateful comments in all directions about the other side. He was inarticulate, and his arguments were disgusting. I came to the conclusion that I was pro-choice but hid my position from Phil because it would have ended our relationship even sooner than it did.

And then there was the issue of home births. They seemed romantic and harkened back to simpler times. However, in my opinion, that era had passed—and for good reason.

And so I had to leave this popular, larger-than-life personality called Phil Shea. I had to say goodbye and forge my own path. There was nothing wrong with either one of us. We were simply incompatible on so many levels.

On looking back, I honestly can't remember the details of the split—amnesia about a traumatic event is a coping strategy—but I'm sure my leaving was done in a clumsy and tearful manner.

I was alone and out on my own now—a solo practitioner.

CHAPTER SIXTEEN
PURSUING EXCELLENCE—
ONE PATIENT AT A TIME

"Hello, Mom. I finally broke up with Dr. Shea. I'm sure that won't come as a big surprise. The end was angry, tearful and complicated. I'm moving into a new office this weekend, and I've been doing a lot of thinking.

"How would you like to be my new receptionist?"

My mother had always wanted to be a nurse, and the idea of helping me and being around patients was—for her—too much to resist. She was: always organized; possessed good people skills; calm under pressure, and had a wisdom and common sense that came from raising her four children.

She jumped at the idea and quit her job at McMaster University where she had worked since Dad's death. My sister, Sandy, agreed to work as a filer, learn how to book patients with specialists, and to schedule tests too. And Mary Jo would serve as the office manager, now that our children were in school.

The next six years until I moved to the United States were the most productive and happiest years of my professional life. My roster swelled. At one point, four female physicians—several of whom had young children at home—rented space in my enlarged office. From there, they could provide care for their small base of patients, see my overflow appointments, and then return home to their waiting families.

The university filmed me interacting with simulated patients—they wanted to use my bedside manner and history-taking technique as a template for medical students to follow. Clinical clerks and nursing students clamored to spend time with me in my practice. The Department of Family Medicine assigned residents to work with me full-time for a year—I was now their Dr. Vince Rudnick. I even made the Canadian College of the Family Physicians finalist list—Family Practice Teacher of the Year—in 1986.

These were heady times.

My life was very typical for a family doctor during that era. There were constant demands and scheduling changes. On any given day, the plan looked like this: hospital rounds first, before my kids were even up; clinic all day; perhaps a house call on the way home; dinner with the family; helping with homework, and then driving to the gym for a late night workout.

However, there was inevitably an emergency: a woman in labor, an on-call night, and meetings to prepare for. 'Turmoil' best described every day.

That and fatigue.

I became an excellent juggler of time. For instance, one Christmas Day that I was on call: I delivered five babies; never missed opening the presents; had brunch at my in-laws, and ate dinner at my mom's. At the time, I felt this was an impressive feat. Now that I'm much older, I recall the details with sadness and regret. Yes, I was in attendance at all those events, but I really wasn't truly present at any one of them.

This type of grueling work schedule was a point of pride when physicians compared notes in the doctors' lounge—all of us gulping coffee—bragging about who had worked more hours the week before. I'm sure that our families weren't proud of who the winner was. They were all at home and wishing we were with them.

It was a gloriously fulfilling professional life. It was also insane and unhealthy on so many levels.

***

It is impossible to tell you about all the patient encounters I've experienced—some mundane, and others bizarre. However, I'd like to share several stories with you that shaped me and, to some extent, changed the course of my life.

The first event involved the Ontario Medical

Association—the OMA—which united physicians in a powerful way. The Association interacted with the provincial government, advocated for improvements in health care, and lobbied for a more favorable fee schedule for physicians.

In general, doctors were unhappy about their shrinking incomes and rising costs. Negotiations with the government became polarized, and an impasse was reached. The OMA signaled that all the physicians might strike if their demands were not met.

A general meeting was called in Toronto, and thousands of Ontario doctors gathered at an enormous convention hall. Our executive team was calling for a work stoppage. They explained that if a strike occurred, only emergency services would be available for patients. That meant I would personally have to close my door.

I could not bear the thought of turning my back on my pregnant patients, who were all due to deliver at any moment. I had promised to be there for them. They had attended my recommended prenatal classes, had a lactation consultant waiting in the wings, and counted on me being present. We had a plan.

What was I supposed to say to them? "Sorry, I'm on strike, and you'll have to go to the hospital and deal with the emergency staff. And, by the way, good luck."

There was no way the OMA was going to keep me from my obstetrical patients, or my patient who was dying at home or, for that matter, any single one of my patients. I was their doctor. We shared an unspoken promise that I would always be there for them, or at least I'd arrange for a trusted associate to be on call if I was away. It would take a much more important issue than a fee schedule dispute to force me to close my door.

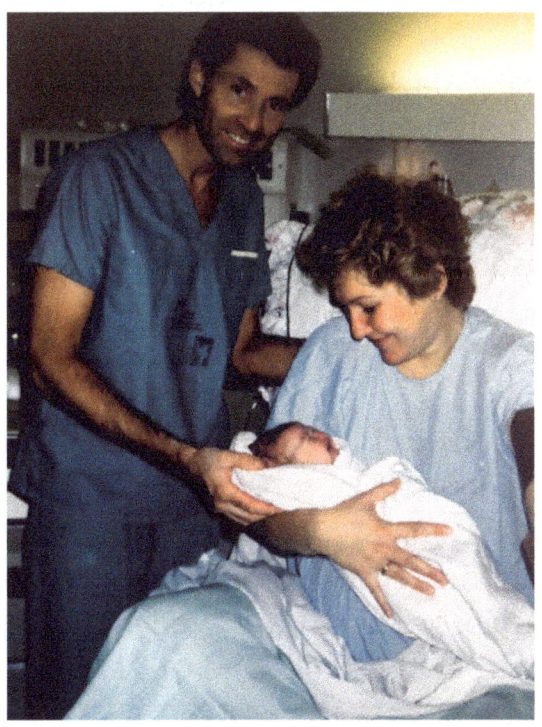

Beatrix and baby David.
Another magical moment for me

I raised my hand at that rancorous OMA meeting and voted NO—there were several others who joined me. Of course the strike took place. It lasted about a week, and I went to work every day. My patients appreciated my commitment to them.

That week, my phone lines were sabotaged. I was threatened by colleagues and called a scab. The provincial government did not budge, and the public turned against the "money-grabbing" doctors. The OMA ultimately called it off, and everyone returned to work. But it took a very long time for fractured relationships to heal.

On looking back, I am proud that I stood up for my principles and honored my obligations to patients. I had learned something about myself—I could be outspoken and brave, and a little obstinate too.

***

The second incident pitted me against the establishment again. It involved the Stevensons, who were long-time patients of mine—I'd delivered their children too. We had a very solid relationship, and they had saved my home phone number from the time when Mrs. S. had been pregnant.

One night at about 1:00 AM, the phone rang. It

was Mr. S. He told me that the fourteen-year old daughter of one of their best friends was in the hospital, and she was close to death. Their friends, along with the Stevensons themselves, were Jehovah's Witnesses, and the daughter was in need of a life-saving blood transfusion. Her parents were refusing treatment, and their doctor had removed himself from the case—claiming that the parents were not cooperating. Mr. S. was hoping that I would consider meeting with the parents and possibly serving as the daughter's attending physician.

He also stressed the immediacy of the situation. Lawyers would be arriving at the hospital for an emergency hearing before Judge Scime at 3:00 AM. Very briefly, the Province was petitioning to have the fourteen year old removed from her parents' authority and made a ward of the provincial government—so the doctors could proceed with transfusions.

It never occurred to me to say no. Something deep inside compelled me to go and at least assess the situation. The Jehovah's Witness congregation was a minority group. They believed in a different ideology and were frequent targets of bullies and the establishment.

I arrived at the hospital at 2:00 AM, introduced myself to the parents, and briefly reviewed the chart. There was a tension—an incredibly hostile atmosphere—that permeated the entire ward.

Apparently, the fourteen year old had been experiencing one of her first menstrual cycles when the bleeding became heavier. It finally became a torrent—soaking pads and towels—and the young lady lost consciousness. She was admitted through emergency to the intensive care unit and assessed by pediatrics, gynecology, hematology, and an intensive care specialist. Intravenous hormone therapy, fluids, and oxygen had been administered, and the bleeding finally stopped. Or perhaps it stopped because she had bled out.

I remember her hemoglobin was 2.8—a number that I had thought was incompatible with life. The physicians were urgently pushing for the transfusions. But the parents reminded them over and over that receiving blood products of any kind was forbidden by their religious beliefs.

The patient was in a room near the nurses' station. I opened the door, and there she was: white as a sheet; oxygen mask in place; hair matted to her scalp; head of the bed down... motionless. Had she died? Her appearance took my breath away.

I introduced myself, and she replied with an almost inaudible voice. Placing my ear literally against her cheek, I asked, "What's your name?"

"Mary."

"Hello, Mary. Your parents asked me to help you. I'm sorry you're so sick. Are you in pain?"

"No."
"Are you scared?"

"No. If I die, I'll go to heaven. Everything will be okay."

"Is your religion important to you?"

"It means everything. It's the best thing about my life."

I was taken aback by her sincerity and her conviction. I told Mary that the hospital doctors wanted to give her a transfusion, and asked how she felt about that.

She became very agitated and said, through clenched teeth, "I'll fight them. I'll tear the intravenous from my arm. How dare they!"

Oh my god! Her breathing became even more rapid and her pulse ridiculously fast. She's going to code. It's going to happen. I held my breath.

I spoke to her in soothing, calming tones, and then promised to help. She slowly surrendered to sleep.

The judicial hearing was just getting started. It was being held in a break room down the hall. I had never attended anything like this before. Her parents sat to one side, and I stopped to let them know I'd be their daughter's new doctor. I took a seat at the front of the room and was the only physician representing the patient. The opposing side was composed of some of the finest specialists in the region—they had been my teachers. We were all sworn in, and the lawyer representing the Province of Ontario passionately presented the case for making this minor—Mary—a ward of the Province. He had an entourage of expert witnesses to bolster his case. Judge Scime took notes.

The judge then turned to me. I testified that the patient was at that very moment a heartbeat away from death. She was on the proverbial razor's edge. Because of the importance of religion in her life, I warned that she would resist a transfusion with all her might…and she would die very quickly from the exertion. My statement was brief and to the point.

Judge Scime adjourned for about fifteen minutes. Once back in session, he ruled quickly. Mary would remain in the care of her parents. There would be no transfusion.

The room emptied rapidly. There were angry stares aimed directly at me. I ignored all of them.

There was no time to waste because I now had the onerous task of serving as Mary's only physician.

To be honest, I was scared. I called several colleagues who gave me invaluable advice about how to hormonally stabilize her uterus and enhance her bone marrow's capacity to make new blood. However, they did not want to become officially involved.

I visited several times a day and encouraged and nurtured Mary in every possible way. Ever so slowly she gained strength. And in a little over a week, my patient was able to walk out of the hospital. I still can't believe she survived.

Once again I was at odds with some of the physicians in the community.

After the incident, they refused to accept my phone calls or referrals. I tried not to let this bother me—but it did. However, I was proud that I had respected and defended another individual's firmly held religious belief. Mary was prepared to die before she would abandon her principles, and I stood right beside her.

Furthermore, I had learned that ordering the "medically correct" therapy could at times be the absolutely wrong thing to do, if you failed to approach the patient holistically. Transfusing this patient would have required restraints and tranquilization. She would have almost certainly died.

These two incidents are etched in my memory. They helped me discover what made me tick and who I really was a person.

However, there were several more adventures just as impactful.

***

My earnings as a cab driver were significant and much higher than my hourly wage as a city worker. When I was a student, I had worked for the Hamilton Streets and Sanitation. It was backbreaking work: loading garbage into a moving truck; cutting weeds in a city park with a scythe; wielding a jackhammer to remove a roadway and expose a broken water main; and scraping and painting miles of old guardrail. However, it was honest labor and allowed me to appreciate how hard my average patient worked to make ends meet.

Now as a family doctor, I was making what I thought was an obscene amount of money. No one in my family had ever been a professional, and they were incapable of providing monetary advice. I was referred to a financial planner—Roger Chilton—by an older physician. Roger proved to be very charismatic and extremely confident. He made certain I had an appropriate amount of life insurance. He also talked about saving so that my children could go to college, and about the best way to plan for my eventual retirement.

Roger devised an aggressive tactic in which I borrowed against the accounts receivable of my practice and the equity in our home. These funds were then invested in limited-partnership products that would allow for incredible returns and tax deductions. I assumed this was how professionals—like doctors, lawyers, dentists—invested for the future.

I trusted the man.

He learned that I had an interest in fast cars and facilitated my purchase of a Porsche. After all, I was working hard and had no time for golf. The car would be an indulgence I could enjoy on a daily basis as I made my rounds.

My colleagues took note of the car and wanted to know how I was doing so well, so I gave them Chilton's number. Word spread, and before you could blink, dozens of physicians had become clients too.

Roger gave us all expensive Christmas gifts and hosted an extravagant yearly party at his mansion near Lake Ontario in Burlington.

Life was good—but not for long.

***

Mandy was a nurse who worked for the Victorian Order of Nurses. The VON provided home care for patients when necessary. I had an enormous roster of devoted patients. At any one time, at least a half dozen of them required this level of care. Since Mandy was assigned to my practice, she visited all my homebound patients and met with me weekly to discuss their status. It was a brilliant arrangement that enhanced good communication and continuity of care.

She was pregnant at the time and asked if I'd accept her as a patient. "Of course," I said, and a few months later I delivered her beautiful baby girl. Another VON nurse covered while she was on maternity leave.

Six months later, Mandy arrived with her infant daughter for a well-baby check and the completion of the first series of immunizations. I noticed that she was limping and asked what had happened. Mandy did not recall an injury. But her left hip was throbbing with pain, and she couldn't securely put weight on it.

Her symptoms did not add up, and I suggested an X ray. The report indicated multiple sites of erosion in her pelvis and proximal femur—highly suggestive of metastatic disease.

You've got to be kidding! Mandy was only in her late twenties—at the beginning of a wonderful life as a wife and mother.

Sure enough, she had an aggressive breast cancer. In a short period of time, and in spite of state-of-the-art chemotherapy, Mandy was confined to home. The bone pain she experienced was intense.

There were no pain experts or palliative-care specialists back in the 1980s, and hospice care was yet to be invented. Her oncologists were of no help either, although one cancer specialist provided some meager prescribing advice by phone.

I was on my own.

Every week, I'd drive from Hamilton to Mandy's home in Burlington—forty minutes—to see how my most recent increased dose of morphine was working. It wasn't. No matter how much I increased the dose, her pain remained uncontrolled. I added a tricyclic antidepressant to augment the narcotic and prescribed anxiolytic and anti-inflammatory medication too. She still experienced terrible pain all over her body—she had metastases everywhere.

My oncologist mentor directed me to increase the morphine dose to absurd numbers. The pharmacy called to verify I really intended to prescribe the indicated amount and to inform me that they were experiencing a shortage that I had caused. But Mandy was still in pain. One morning, her husband called my office and demanded that I visit immediately. Patient appointments were cancelled, and I exceeded the speed limit to get to their home as soon as possible. I could hear chiming from the bell tower of a nearby church as I exited my car.

I had never seen this before. Mandy's head had blown up like a balloon. Her face was purple, and her strikingly blue eyes were almost obscured by periorbital edema. She had developed superior vena cava syndrome because the cancer had spread inside her upper chest. It was now blocking blood from exiting her head. Her distress was palpable.

Mandy's husband grabbed my shoulders and stared angrily into my eyes as he said, "Do something! Quit screwing around! Do something! This is intolerable!"

After I administered every last bit of medicine in their household, Mandy finally settled down. She expired several hours later.

I had utterly failed—for many weeks—to alleviate

her distress, and vowed to learn more about pain management in the future. This was not an idle promise. I never wanted to experience a palliative-care debacle like this ever again.

Please forgive me, Mandy.

***

The red-faced man burst into the office and yelled that his wife was in labor. He pleaded for help. The couple had been on their way to the hospital when they realized they wouldn't make it—the baby was coming too fast. They saw my office sign, took a chance and pulled into the lot. He was frantic.

My mom—the receptionist—grabbed me from an exam room, and we raced to a car that was parked cock-eyed near the entrance door. A pregnant woman was in the back seat, naked from the waist down, and she was in an advanced stage of labor. There was no time for introductions.

Mom appeared with a wheelchair, and once inside an examination room, we lifted the panting lady onto the table. I hurriedly gathered my recently retired home birth bag, while Mom corralled towels, sheets, gowns, and boiled the proverbial water.

Both Sandy and Mom fetched whatever was needed. My reception area became a labor-and-delivery waiting room as patients arrived for appointments and became caught up in the excitement. Everyone held their collective breath. Then they heard a cry—tiny at first—and then a fullthroated wail.

I could hear applause coming from the waiting room. I peeked out the door to discover that everyone was standing and clapping. "It's a boy!" I said. My mother beamed—you would have thought her new grandson had been born. She was so proud of me and how I had performed

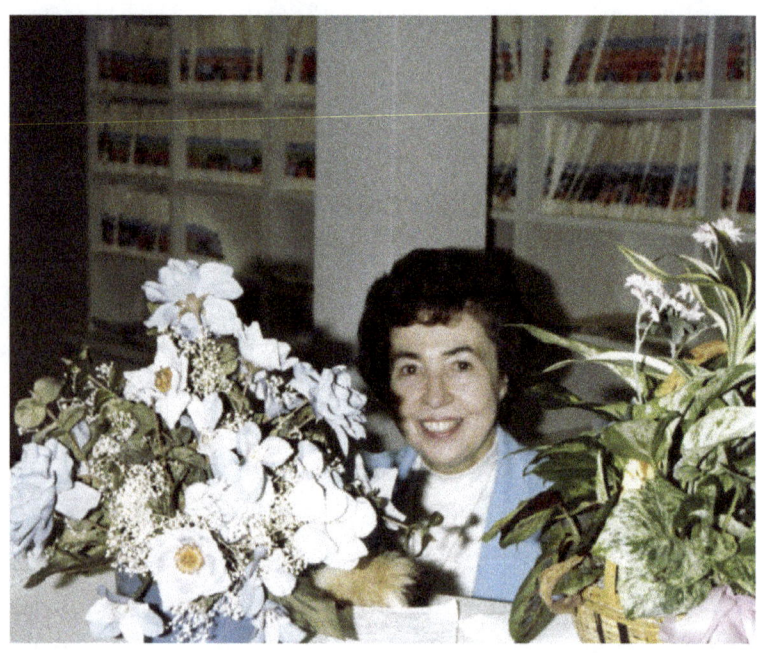

Mom—the receptionist—and her flowers

during this crisis. It was the best day of her entire work career.

The new father insisted on taking photos of everyone involved. About an hour later, while I was seeing my regularly scheduled patients, the happy couple with their healthy baby left the office. Mom and Sandy helped them to their car. The new mom had not required stitches, and they never did go to the hospital.

The husband returned to the office the next day, bearing gifts and flowers for Mom and Sandy. The couple lived out of town and we didn't have their insurance information; it wasn't worth the hassle, and I never pursued billing them.

I had been paid in full with their gratitude, which further confirmed that I was a lousy businessman.

Perhaps this was the reason for my participation in home births over all those many years. It had prepared me perfectly for this moment in time.

And now I could tell the story of this office birth for the rest of my career.

***

My resident was busy seeing a patient, and I was about to enter another examination room when I heard something about the stock market from the waiting room television. I stopped and listened. It was Monday, October 19, 1987, and the DOW had just fallen 508 points—the largest one-day drop in history, percentage wise. That day became known as Black Monday. And while I didn't realize it at the time, the events that followed would change my life forever.

At the end of the day, I called Roger Chilton for reassurance. He sounded excited and talked about what a wonderful opportunity this was. He said I should think about investing even more aggressively in the next couple of days.

"Calm down," he said. "Everything is going to be great. You worry too much. You're going to be a rich man someday, Dr. Bob Lancaster."

I didn't believe a word he said.

***

There are so many more medical stories to tell. How about the burly, fearless police officer—a beat cop—who had just lost his wife to diabetic complications. He and his nine year old son were grief-stricken, and now he had chest pain. His electrocardiogram indicated that a heart attack was in process, and he refused an ambulance. He would not go to the hospital unless I came with him—he was scared. He begged, and against my better judgment, I drove him from my office to

The Doctor Is In

the emergency department. My receptionist called ahead, and the staff was waiting as I screeched to a stop. I'm certain none of my colleagues would have done something this stupid—or perhaps they have their own ridiculous stories too. I held his hand as he was whisked away to the coronary care unit. He survived and continued his career, this time behind a desk.

***

What about the father who refused to look at his newborn son? The baby obviously had Down syndrome. There had not been any prenatal genetic screening, and the diagnosis had caught everyone by surprise. Not only that, he said he wanted the child placed for adoption, and forbade his wife to see the baby. The mother was hospitalized for several days while she recovered from her Cesarean section, and the father was shunned by the staff. Of course I still visited and held the baby in the nursery—we spent fifteen minutes every day in the rocking chair together.

On the third day post-partum, I was seated at the nurses' station late that evening. I had just attended another delivery and was writing a note when I felt a tap on my shoulder. It was the father—he wanted to see his son. He asked if I would take him because he felt hated by the staff and needed my support.

I retrieved the baby from the bassinet, found a quiet corner in the nursery, and presented the tiny bundle to this new father. We looked at the little guy from top to bottom, and I pointed out how beautiful his baby was. To make a long story short, Dad bonded with his son that night. The family left the hospital together the next morning, and this man became one of the most loving parents I have ever had the privilege to know.

Perhaps I've said enough. By now, I think you've come to better understand the life of a busy family physician. One minute you're soaring with the angels—having just been part of a magical patient experience. The next thing you know, your heart is being ripped out by an unbelievably sad turn of events for an unlucky family.

CHAPTER SEVENTEEN
STORMY DAYS

With the luxury of hindsight, I'm going to stop the clock in 1990, and take stock of my life—both professional and personal. At this point, I'd been in practice for ten years. The trials and tribulations of medical school, clerkship, and residency were a distant memory. However, all that hard work had allowed me to become a skilled family physician.

Professionally, one of my biggest strengths involved my communication skills. I had mastered the art of an effective bedside manner, which included the ability to empathize, explain, and motivate. Patients sensed within a few seconds that they had my full attention and that I cared—because I really did care. They did not feel rushed, and we could cover a lot of ground in one visit. I also had discovered I had this uncanny ability to diagnose a patient's symptoms, even those that had stumped many other clinicians. As a result of these strengths, I was highly sought after and had amassed a huge roster of patients.

My office was truly a family-run enterprise, with no daily melodrama. Most often it was business-as-usual, which included a mountain of paperwork and multiple daily fights with OHIP to obtain care for a patient.

The provincial government controlled all things related to health care, including: doctors' fee schedules; the number of hospital and nursing home beds; the availability of special tests, like cardiac catheterizations and CT scans; a preferred medication formulary; the size of a medical school class; the number of internship and residency positions—to name but a few.

Since the provincial government controlled the purse strings, every aspect of the provision of care was underfunded. Yes, all the citizenry had health insurance, but when they actually needed care, they were usually placed on a list where they would wait, and wait some more.

It was becoming increasingly more difficult for me to admit really sick patients to the hospital. Instead they would languish in emergency, waiting for a hospital bed to be vacated—sometimes for days. At times there was a line of gurneys—each one occupied by someone quite ill—out the door of the emergency room and down a hallway. The sought-after medical beds, within the hospital proper, were often occupied by patients who simply could not be discharged, because they had dementia or whatever. They were waiting for a nursing home bed to open up, except there were no beds—another example of underfunding.

The whole system functioned like a game of

musical chairs, and the government had removed far too many chairs. Patients and their families were frustrated and impatient. They demanded action, and their powerless family physicians—like me—were caught in the middle and the recipients of their rage. The situation was intolerable.

And then there was the issue of money. Because of the professional success of my practice, I was generating an income that was dizzying when compared to my cab-driver earnings. My father had passed away in 1984. However, even if he were still alive, advising me on the financial aspects of my life would have been well beyond his comfort zone—and mine too. Naively, I had turned everything over to Roger Chilton, and his grand investment scheme had imploded. The stock market crash of 1987 had been a seminal event, and a number of awful things followed, including the collapse of the housing market. Lenders became nervous and demanded immediate repayment of loans because the value of leveraged assets—items like our beautiful home—had shrunk considerably. And Revenue Canada had disallowed the promised tax deductibility of all of Chilton's recommended limited-partnership investments.

There is nothing more sobering than a large, unexpected tax bill and a margin call from the bank. And it wasn't just me, either.

All of Chilton's physician clients experienced severe financial stress. To my knowledge, the entire bunch of us declared bankruptcy at some point in time—all except two. One family physician embarked on a long legal battle. The other, an internist in a nearby small town, committed suicide.

Now I'll turn my attention to the state of my personal life.

I've come to the conclusion that exposing a person like me, with my strong care-giver personality, to a large group of people who need help is akin to placing an alcoholic in a job selling alcohol.

The patients are so thankful for the care they receive. They sing your praises, ply you with presents, and send their family and friends to you. This is very heady stuff! However, for me it was also a trap. I'd become addicted to work—and to all the wonderful accolades and thanks I received on a daily basis. At the same time, I was neglecting my family. Oh, I was there for the kids' birthday parties, swim meets, and big events. But I wasn't with them for those long lazy days in which we could simply hang out. I somehow found time to rock other parents' babies in the hospital nursery, but I was unable to find the time to hold my own children.

What little free time I had was spent mowing our

two-acre lawn and trimming the bushes. It's easy to assume that I was too cheap to hire help. In reality, I was a perfectionist—a micro-manager—and no one could do the landscaping as well as me. And hadn't I received two Trillium Awards from the Royal Botanical Gardens as proof of my horticultural skills?! Need I tell you who also removed the snow from our four-hundred-foot driveway in the winter?

The rest of my leisure time was devoted to maintaining my once formidable competitive golf game, some degree of physical fitness—and crying. That's correct. I cried a lot, especially when I was alone and had nothing scheduled. I'd think of Bobbi. Yes, I still identified as a female, and the yearning to be myself was overwhelming at times. I felt trapped and could not imagine a path forward in which I could lead a truly authentic life.

The end result was that Mary Jo and I were leading parallel lives. Given my absence, her interests revolved around the children and the special needs that Jeff presented. Somewhere along the way, the pilot light of our marriage had blown out.

You might assume that my professional and personal issues were unique to me—if so, you would be dead wrong. Yes, my gender dysphoria was an additional issue. Otherwise, most of my colleagues across the province looked a lot like me.

Our training at McMaster—as forward-thinking as it was—did not provide us with any meaningful guidance in these matters. This meant that we were an at-risk population for many untoward outcomes, including: depression; suicide; family dysfunction; divorce; alcoholism; drug abuse; sexual impropriety, and more. And it's not like these were theoretical possibilities—they were happening all around, with tragic consequences.

Thousands of Canadian physicians came up with a solution they thought would solve everything. They moved to the United States and enjoyed a fresh start. Several colleagues within my social circle left for Arizona, and word trickled back home about how well they were doing. It was a tantalizing solution. Mary Jo and I had visited that enchanting desert landscape on two prior occasions; we dreamed of retiring there someday. And yet, we were just forty years old and nowhere close to retirement age. However, now maybe was the time?

We talked endlessly about the pros and cons of uprooting: the challenge of a new school system for the children; clearing immigration; finding work; becoming licensed, and the reality of being far away from our respective families.

Much to the dismay of her parents and my mom, Mary Jo and I decided to leave. I promised in the future to be more present at home, which meant: curtailing my practice size, doing fewer calls, and giving up the very family-disruptive activity of delivering babies.

Mary Jo and I were going to be a real team. The year was 1991. Maybe somewhere during this new adventure, we'd fall in love all over again.

… Doctor Is In

CHAPTER EIGHTEEN
GREENER PASTURES

A former Hamilton patient—Valerie—had managed to track me down in Arizona and left a message with my new receptionist in Phoenix. It was imperative she speak with me as soon as possible. What in the world was this going to be about?

It was my first week seeing patients in my new office in sunny Phoenix—115 degrees outside. Words cannot truly describe all the hurdles I had overcome during this transition to a new country: securing a green card; passing license exams; selling my Hamilton practice; listing our Scenic Drive home; establishing business and personal accounts with a bank. And I was also adjusting to being alone, because Mary Jo and the children were still back in Hamilton—finishing their school year and packing. Every which way I turned, there was: another document to sign, hospital privilege forms, accountant statements, an apartment lease, a car purchase, brokerage contracts, promissory notes, new credit cards—the list was endless.

"Hello, Valerie. It's Dr. Lancaster. Is everything alright?"

"Thanks for calling back. My family is okay. We

were saddened to learn you moved to Arizona because we don't think we will ever experience a doctor like you again. However, I was horrified to read that Dr. Johnson had taken over your practice."

"Do you know Dr. Johnson? Tell me more."

"He was my doctor before I switched to you. This is awkward to tell you about. He touched me in a sexual way during one of my visits, and he made a suggestive comment. I was repulsed and never saw the creep again. I mentioned the incident to several girlfriends who had visited his family-practice office too. They recounted a similar experience and had ditched him as well. I thought you should know."

I thanked Valerie for the information, and we said our goodbyes.

Her story was very believable, and it made me sick. What kind of predator had I unwittingly given access to my beloved patients back home?

Even though I was in the middle of a very chaotic move, I returned home to meet with Dr. Johnson. I was prepared to return his practice purchase money and to find a safe harbor for my old patients.

We met at his residence, and his wife immediately

inserted herself. She did not allow me to get a word in edgewise. Mrs. Johnson said she was appalled that I had accused her husband of sexual impropriety. She knew her husband better than any other person on earth, and argued he was incapable of this alleged behavior. He was a good man, a loving husband, and how dare I sully his character!

Mrs. Johnson was a force to be reckoned with. I apologized and wished them good luck. At least the trip was an opportunity to see Mary Jo and the kids.

***

I returned to Phoenix where I continued to familiarize myself with a complicated system involving multiple insurance companies. My new staff could not have been more helpful. The retiring doctor was not much older than me. However, he was seriously depressed, and his mood worried us all.

My schedule required me to see fewer patients than in a typical workday back home, and billing for three times the money. My office expenses were less; I could order any test, and it would be done the next day. The specialists were welcoming and top notch, and the family-practice teaching unit next door requested I become involved as a preceptor. There was no doubt—

The Doctor Is In

I had died and gone to heaven.

During my idle time, I researched the best schools in Phoenix; hunted for a suitable family home; investigated swim teams for Laura; explored special education for Jeff, and located a terrific piano teacher for Jennifer. And then I retreated to my little apartment. One night, I heard gunshots in the courtyard and peeked out the curtains to observe a SWAT team in action. Well, what else did I expect? I was living in the United States of America—the land of the free and the home of the brave.

This alone time provided something else too. I could be Bobbi—at least within the confines of my meager rental space. It was exhilarating to at least have one toe out of the closet.

***

Mary Jo and the children arrived in the fall of 1991, just in time to start the school year. We purchased an incredible home at an extremely low price in toney Paradise Valley. Arizona had also experienced a collapse of its real estate market, which made the house affordable. Mary Jo once again became my office manager, and the original physician exited the scene and moved to Oregon. Several years later, I learned that he had died of an accidental overdose.

We explored every inch of Arizona as a family. We enjoyed Alaskan and Mexican cruises; a vacation in Hawaii, and a houseboat adventure on Lake Powell in northern Arizona too.

For a brief period of time, I joined a Canadian group of family physicians until we parted ways for even greener pastures. Practicing medicine in the States quickly became more challenging with the emergence of something called HMOs. And many hospital organizations were purchasing practices to secure a patient base that would continue to feed their hospital. The physicians were given handsome salaries—including me. There were corporate mergers, consolidations, buy-outs and bankruptcies. The physicians were bought and sold like stocks, and each new acquisition required moving the practice to a different corporate location.

During one of these disruptions, my mother called from Hamilton with some disturbing news. Dr. Johnson had been charged with sexual assault involving a patient. He had made the front page and eventually was found guilty and given considerable jail time. This made me sick. Perhaps I should have done more a few years earlier. Maybe I could have called the College of Physician and Surgeons—the licensing body—and reported what my patient had told me.

***

On paper, Mary Jo and I had emerged unscathed from our personal bankruptcy. We had survived the enormous stress involved in immigrating to a new country. Our house was beautiful; the girls were enrolled in a top college preparatory school; Jeff was receiving excellent special education, and I had attained a better work-life balance.

There was only one thing missing—a little thing called love. Try as we might, Mary Jo and I could not reignite the spark our marriage once had. It was over, and we were done. Yes, my gender dysphoria contributed. However, there were a dozen other reasons that are no one else's business.

The purpose of this book is to chronicle my medical adventures from start to finish. I do not want to stray too far from that theme and get lost in the personal dramas that unfold in every life. However, I've already listed the problems that physicians in general were at risk of experiencing. If you are keeping score, I was gradually checking all the boxes.

Exposing my personal life to all of you is not easy. However, if even one reader seeks help and avoids a disaster because I have exposed the pitfalls, then it has all been worthwhile.

I left my marriage much like I'd left Dr. Shea: clumsily, with lots of tears, and a dollop of brief anger for added effect. Our divorce was not adversarial—we shared the same lawyer. Mary Jo and I didn't hate each other. On the contrary, we had three teenage children who needed our full attention.

Unfortunately, my mother-in-law finally had something tangible to hate me for. She erased my image from every family photo and boasted that she knew all along that I would leave her daughter when we moved far away.

Now how could she have known that, even before we were aware of our problems? And why had she not lifted a finger to warn us or help?

The Doctor Is In

CHAPTER NINETEEN
GONE TOO SOON

We met at work in the fall of 1995. Lucy was a nurse practitioner who was hired by a hospital organization to help care for my large roster of patients. She was well trained, and at one time had been a critical-care nurse and a clinical nurse educator at Brigham and Women's Hospital in Boston.

This was her first foray into family medicine. She was eager to learn, and I would be her mentor. The situation was reminiscent of when I supervised McMaster family-medicine residents many years ago in Hamilton.

I was teaching again.

Lucy reminded me that she was an educator too, and we traded talking points and approaches. She also made it clear that she worked for the hospital—she was not my nurse practitioner—and her years of training were equal to mine. Lucy was, and is, a force to be reckoned with. She introduced me to nursing concepts, which are much more patient-centric. My training had been disease-focused. It took a while for me to realize that the script had been flipped, and I was actually the learner.

Lucy was most impressed with my bedside manner, the time I took with patients, and my explanations. She expressed surprise at my gentle, caring nature—unusual in her many years of dealing with hospital staff physicians. At one point, Lucy paid me the ultimate compliment. She said, "Dr. Lancaster… you would have been a tremendous nurse."

We made hospital rounds and house calls together. We also attended medical education courses and events sponsored by pharmaceutical companies. Given the long work days, Lucy and I got to know each other very well in a short period of time.

The best care we provided revolved around an unusual group of patients. Allow me to explain.

An internist in central Phoenix looked after a large number of gay men who had contracted HIV and were struggling with AIDS. However, the physician could not find anyone to sign out to when he needed a break. This was a time of ignorance and fear, even within the healthcare community.

Given my own closeted life—living with the worry that somebody might find out—I could smell discrimination a mile away. And this internist and his patients were being ostracized. I connected with the physician and agreed to be on call for him.

And then the unthinkable happened. This caring doctor, who ministered to a marginalized community, experienced a brain hemorrhage. He survived but was extremely damaged, and would require nursing-home-level treatment for the rest of his life.

The manager of his practice was distraught. And now she couldn't find anyone to take over his practice. I told her I would be honored to take his patients in. However, I did not have a clue about the management of AIDS.

Lucy really stepped up. Together, we contacted an AIDS expert—took him to lunch—and asked every conceivable question. We read everything we could get our hands on and became experts around the management of this most complicated group of patients.

These gay men were a riot. Of course they were ill. But they were also outrageous, flamboyant, outspoken and beautiful human beings—professional dancers, artists, hairdressers—who you couldn't help but fall in love with.

In spite of our best efforts, they all died. Their deaths were horrible: disfiguring cancers; disgusting sores; unrelenting coughing, and weight loss that reduced them to skeletons. One minute they were vibrant individuals in the prime of their life, and then they were gone.

We accepted other AIDS patients, too. Most memorable was a preteen African–American, Sasha, who had contracted the illness *in utero*. Her father doted on her and attended every visit. She was smart; full of life; had a big smile, and she always styled her hair using multiple randomly placed pigtails.

One weekend, Sasha became very ill and was seen and discharged from two emergency departments. Early Monday morning, she and her father were waiting outside our locked clinic door. Sasha was slumped forward in a wheelchair—we represented their last hope. I was rounding on hospital patients and was oblivious to her plight. However, Lucy was inside the clinic when the doors opened and Sasha took her last breath.

She collapsed and coded in the examination room. Lucy attended to her immediately. No one in the clinic was more experienced at resuscitation than Lucy. She had participated on countless arrest teams throughout her career and had even taught CPR and Advanced Life Support. Sasha was unconscious but still alive when the paramedics transferred her to the emergency department.

The Doctor Is In

The overhead public address in the hospital announced my name, requesting that I call the switchboard. That was the moment I learned of Sasha's crisis, and I hurried to emergency. I arrived in time to hear the arrest team call off the code—she was gone. The only thing left to do was console her father.

When I arrived at the office, an internist, who also worked in the multidisciplinary clinic, took me aside and literally screamed at me. He said Lucy and I had no business welcoming these AIDS patients into our space and placing him and the staff at risk. He was certain the management of this disease belonged in the hands of specialists—we should stick to our job of being gate-keepers.

Of course, he had no idea just how much encouragement and training we had received from two infectious disease experts—both of whom were overwhelmed by the epidemic. They were thrilled that at least some primary care providers were willing to step forward and be part of the solution, too.

This arrogant internist made an already terrible situation even uglier, and I'll never forget his insensitivity.

The Doctor Is In

CHAPTER TWENTY
THE HEART OF THE MATTER

I'm sure that you could see this coming. Lucy and I fell in love and were married in May 1999. It was a second marriage for both of us, and we were committed to making this work. We promised to help each other to be the best version of ourselves that we could be. Our mutual devotion, affection and admiration were noted by many friends. Some commented wistfully that they wished they had the magic in their relationship that we had obviously found in ours.

By this time, the hospital-owned clinic where we met had collapsed—another failed corporate initiative. Lucy found work in a family medicine clinic in Gilbert, and I was employed by yet another hospital-run clinic in Phoenix.

Initially, the cracks were barely visible. I was fifty years old and having difficulty seeing as many people a day as was expected. There was an irritability and impatience within me, and I was more easily distracted. My enthusiasm for helping people had not waned. However, I missed my old solo practice in Hamilton.

We moved to the small town of Gold Canyon to simplify our life and reduce monthly expenses. This little village reminded us both of our childhood homes. I found work in a local clinic, and later established a concierge-style house call practice. Lucy and I were on solid ground, or so I thought.

At this point, those little cracks were becoming harder to hide. I began to ruminate about all my past failures and the damage my decisions had caused. Leaving Mary Jo was at the top of the list. How could I have broken my promise "to have and to hold, until death do us part?" The repercussions felt by our children, as a result of the divorce, were real and painful too.

Aside from this, there was the bankruptcy. How could I have been so foolish to choose an incompetent financial planner all those many years ago? And what about selling my Hamilton practice to a sexual predator? Even the decision to move to Arizona was on the table. Perhaps I should have stayed in Canada, accepted the fact I was going to lose our house to creditors, weathered the embarrassment, and carried on. I missed my old patients. I felt badly about the manner in which I'd left Dr. Shea. And, as ridiculous as this appears, I even wondered if my eighth-grade classmate, who I'd promised to take to a dance, had ever forgiven me—I had failed to honor my commitment and never did call her back.

All of these issues weighed me down, and I

obsessed about them constantly. And then I shared my cross-dressing and gender concerns with Lucy. After her initial curiosity, she made it absolutely clear that this behavior was unwelcome and a non-starter.

My private crying occurred almost daily.

***

I sense you're getting restless and are collectively asking the question, "What happened to that engaging book that was supposed to talk about the professional adventures of a McMaster medical school graduate?" Well, this graduate was sick, and time was running out.

It was depression—pervasive, severe, and potentially lethal. In fact, I finally decided to kill myself. My suicide plan was well-organized, and the method was going to be precise. Would you have expected anything less?

And then Lucy discovered my hidden letters addressed to all who mattered. They were all in envelopes—addressed and stamped—ready to be mailed the next day. Sensing that something wasn't right, she had gone snooping through my briefcase and desk.

Then all hell broke loose! Before I could blink, I was brought to my family doctor's office. This was followed by a psychiatrist, psychologists, therapists, medication, and counseling for several years.

After a chaotic time, further complicated by a stroke, the fundamental issue—the crux of the matter—had become obvious. I was transgender, and any hope of survival and a meaningful recovery revolved around self-acceptance and living my life openly.

***

The process of transitioning and becoming Bobbi started in my mid-fifties, and it was unimaginably complicated for me and all concerned. However, from the moment the decision was made, I felt relieved. In fact, my face often hurt from smiling—something I was doing a lot more of.

Perhaps it was no coincidence that exciting opportunities came my way almost immediately. Aside from my small house-call practice, I became the medical director of two inpatient rehabilitation facilities. I was about to learn a great deal about a field I did not know much about.

At the same time, I accepted a position as one of the medical directors of an enormous hospice company in Phoenix. My duties included making house calls on terminally ill patients and supporting them and their families. They lived in and around my home, many on farms or in trailer parks. The work allowed me to interact with amazing palliative care nurses, social workers, and pastoral care staff. I was required to complete many courses. My knowledge and abilities on the treatment of pain and other terminal symptoms grew exponentially.

Unfortunately, my expertise in this area of palliative care came twenty years too late to help Mandy—my beloved VON nurse, young mother and victim of a particularly aggressive breast cancer.

By 2012, I was at the zenith of my career—happy, fulfilled, and proud of the level of care I was providing. My performance reviews were extremely positive, and I was cherished by the staff at all the facilities I served.

It was time to discuss my impending social transition with my private patients and my employers. They didn't know it yet, but they were about to meet Dr. Bobbi Lancaster.

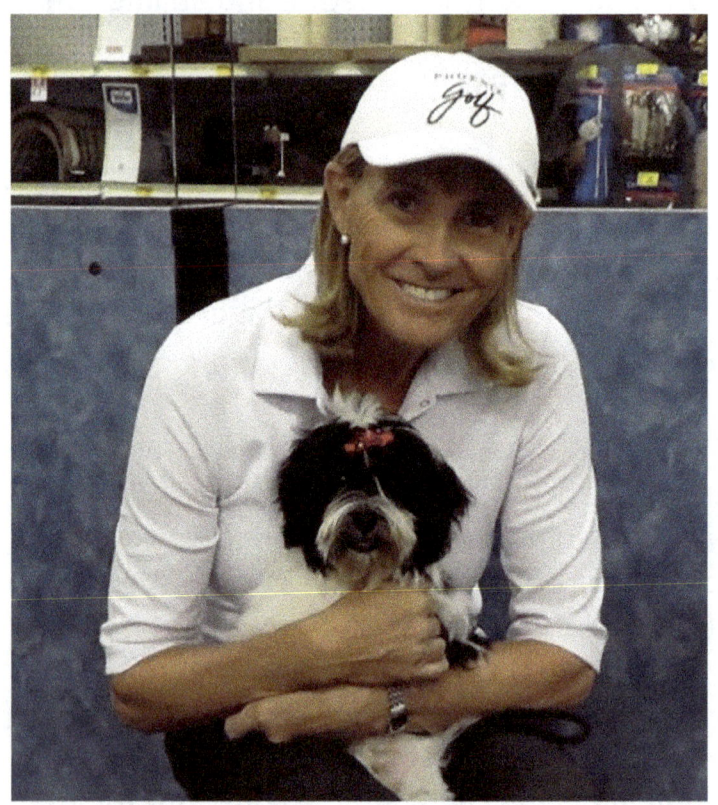

Bobbi and Bentley

CHAPTER TWENTY-ONE
ADVOCACY

Have you ever lived in fear of being fired? Do you remember staring at the ceiling—unable to sleep—as you wondered how you would pay the bills when your employment was terminated? Was there ever a time when your heart was ripped out of your chest and you were left on the curb of life, like a piece of unwanted garbage?

All of these terrible events happened to me.

First, I met with Dr. Owens, the executive medical director of the hospice company. He listened to my transgender story, and learned about the changes everyone was about to see. He heard how much I enjoyed serving as one of their directors, and of my desire to continue in that role as Dr. Bobbi.

Dr. Owens remained poker-faced. There would be deliberations and discussions—meetings that never happened. Nothing derogatory was ever said. However, over the next several months—while I tossed and turned in my bed—his veiled decision was made public. Dr. Owens announced that the company had decided to stop serving the rural area where I lived and saw patients. "It was a cost-saving decision," he said. Unfortunately, there were no other positions for me in the organization, and I was gone.

Within a few months, I learned they had hired another primary care provider to minister to hospice patients in my old geographical area. It was blatantly obvious that letting me go had nothing to do with saving money. Dr. Owens had found a way to get rid of me, without looking like he was discriminating against a transgender employee.

In reality, his elaborate scheme was unnecessary because Arizona is a right-to-work state, and a person can be fired without justification. Furthermore, there are no anti-discrimination laws in Arizona that protect transgender individuals like me. Dr. Owens could do whatever he wanted to do. And he did.

Simultaneously, I met with Mr. Cullen—the owner of the rehabilitation company. He had actually arranged the meeting, and that in itself was unusual. Up to that point, Mr. Cullen had been very pleased with my performance as medical director. However, I discovered he had been alerted by a member of the staff, who had observed some changes in me that were difficult to hide: long hair, ear-piercings, and my growing breasts that were impossible to completely camouflage—even with the use of a binder and over-sized shirt. This senior employee had figured out what was going on, and reported to the owner. Now Mr. Cullen wanted to observe me first-hand.

From the outset, I noticed the owner's demeanor had changed—he'd become cold. I didn't dare bring up being transgender. Mr. Cullen was a devoted Mormon, and I sensed his religious beliefs were now determining my future. Given that I had lost my hospice job, I was really worried about being let go a second time.

A few weeks went by, and I continued to present myself as Dr. Bob. However, it was becoming more difficult to hide the physical changes that hormones and surgery had caused. It became painfully obvious that I was going to have to meet with Mr. Cullen again.

I never got the chance.

One morning, I arrived for work at the rehabilitation center to discover my office had been completely rearranged, and my desk was nowhere to be found. The secretary—who shared the space—turned away from my puzzled gaze, and began to cry. I recall standing in place, completely confused. Then I saw the manager walking toward the office. She presented me with a cardboard box that contained my stethoscope, a spider plant, prescription pads, a photo of Lucy, reference books, and several other personal items.

"I'm sorry," she said. "We've decided to hire a new medical director, because the owner wants to take the company in a new direction." I slinked out the front door—in front of the staff—and held the box close to my chest, in an effort to hide my humiliation.

Thankfully, my private patients stuck with me—they could not imagine losing me their personal physician—no matter what I looked like. Nevertheless, Lucy and I found ourselves in a serious financial situation.

What to do?

Should I proceed with legal action—with the help of the ACLU or Lambda Legal—and be the plaintiff in a landmark discrimination case that might eventually wend its way to the Supreme Court? It would feel good to punish my employers for the cavalier way in which they had thrown me aside. My dismissal at both companies had nothing to do with my performance. It was clearly because I was transgender. Revenge would be sweet. However, the thought of taking legal action made me feel dirty. I feared I would begin to see myself as a victim and be consumed by a protracted adversarial process.

Out of fairness, I spent considerable time thinking about the conundrum I'd presented for my employers. I had blind-sided them. They'd hired me, in good faith, as Dr. Bob—a male. For multiple reasons, I was the perfect fit for their business. There was no way to warn them about the future because when they contracted with me, I was still not clear about my future either. Once my transition became a reality, how could I criticize them for rejecting me? In their eyes, I had misrepresented myself—albeit unintentionally. I could see why they felt deceived or betrayed.

So once again, I was back at the starting point. Should I hire a bunch of lawyers and take everyone to task? Or should I step back, take a breath and do something fun—like playing tournament golf again? I certainly had free time on my hands, and wondered if I could still compete with the same level of skill as when I was younger. For me the decision was obvious.

I went golfing.

After dusting off my clubs I requested permission to compete as a female—in accordance with a gender policy that had been developed by the United States Golf Association. Once granted, I quickly won two tournaments against highly skilled amateur players. There were derogatory comments made that I had an unfair advantage.

"She hits the ball too far because she was once a man," was a frequently heard complaint.

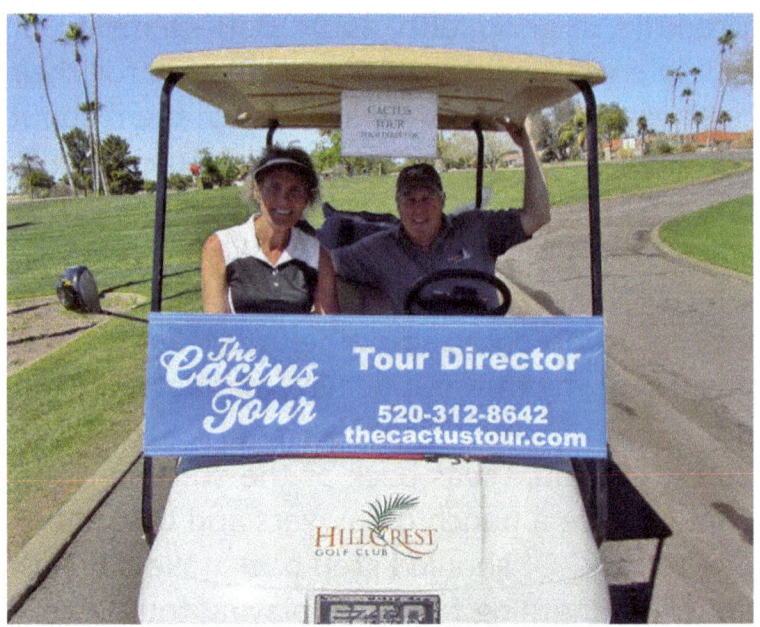

Me and Mike Brown, the tour director

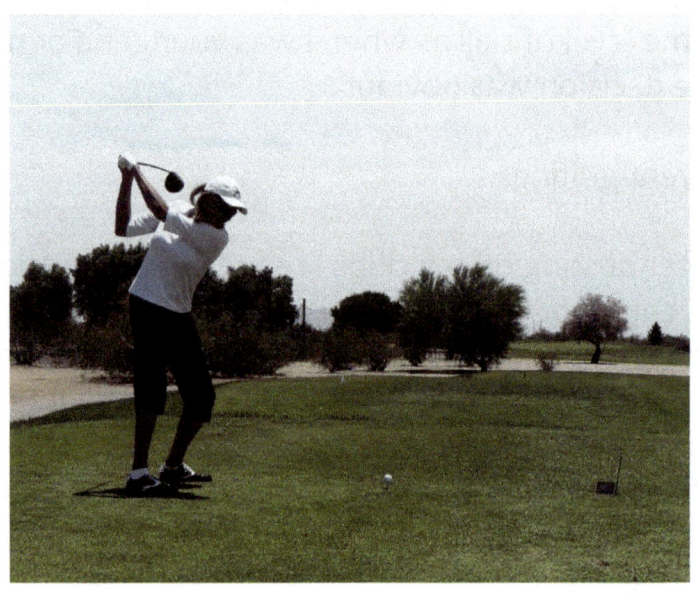

Pounding another 270-yard drive

To avoid being called a cheat, I withdrew from amateur events and competed on the Cactus Tour against elite athletes—forty years younger than me. No one could accuse me of having an unfair physical advantage now.

I'd always wanted to be a professional golfer. I might have been sixty-three years old, but I was able to hold my own. My best finish was third place in an event in Apache Junction, Arizona.

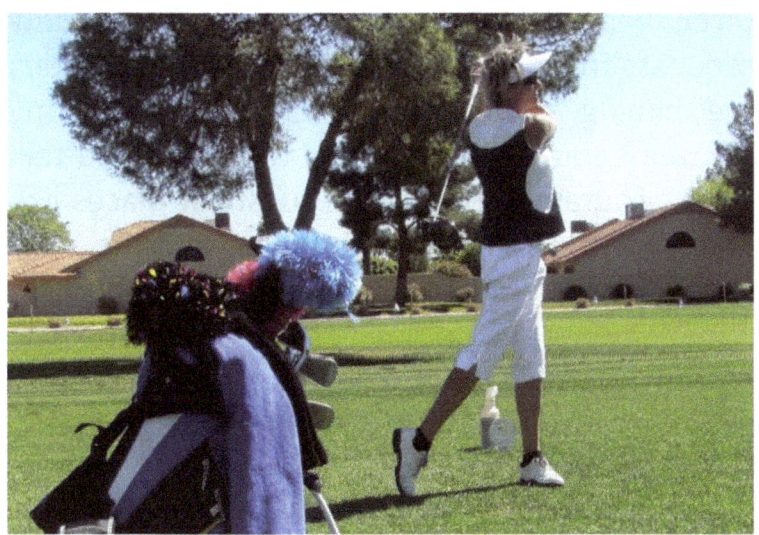

Nice form!

One thing led to another, and I attempted to qualify for the LPGA Tour. I competed in their qualifying tournament at Palm Springs, California, in August of 2013.

I have documented these events in my memoir, *The Red Light Runner*. Suffice it to say that I did not qualify for the LPGA. However, I did secure status on the second most prestigious tour in the world—the Symetra Tour. And then an unexpected thing happened along the way. The media became intrigued by my story: a transgender woman; sixty-three years old; a family physician; attempting to become a world-class professional golfer.

My life changed quite abruptly. During the next three years, there were dozens of interview requests from national and international media; the filming of four documentaries about my life; appearances on national television and talk radio programs; speaking requests at places like Stanford, the University of Kansas and the Weill Cornell Medical Center in New York; numerous engagements at community colleges and medical schools; participation in a White House Summit concerning myriad transgender issues; election to the national board of directors of the Human Rights Campaign; lobbying on Capitol Hill for transgender rights and equality, as well as participation on many panels and in several debates. I received multiple awards for my human rights advocacy, including: the treasured Equality Award from HRC; induction into the Echo Magazine Hall of Fame, and election to the McMaster University Alumni Gallery—McMaster's Hall of Fame.

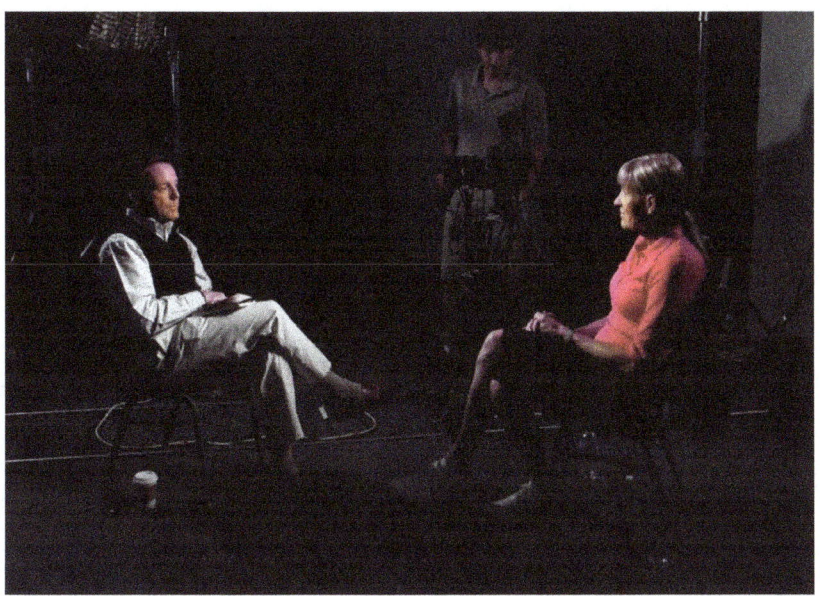

NBC Sportscaster Jimmy Roberts interviews me on the Golf Channel

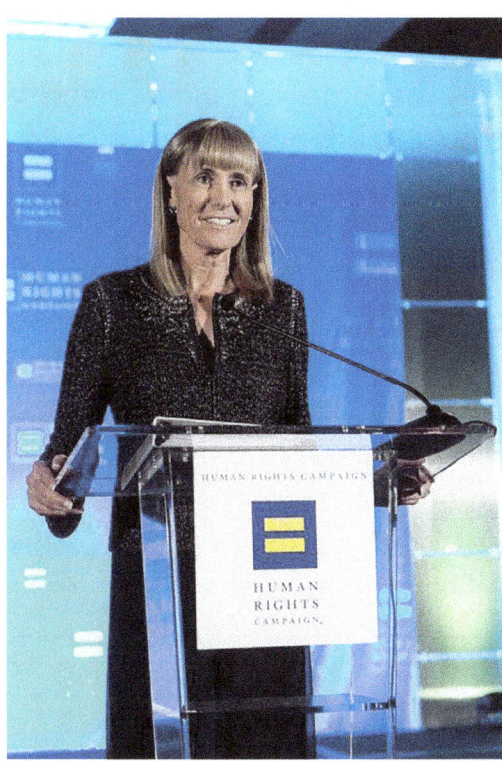

Speaking about equality and acceptance

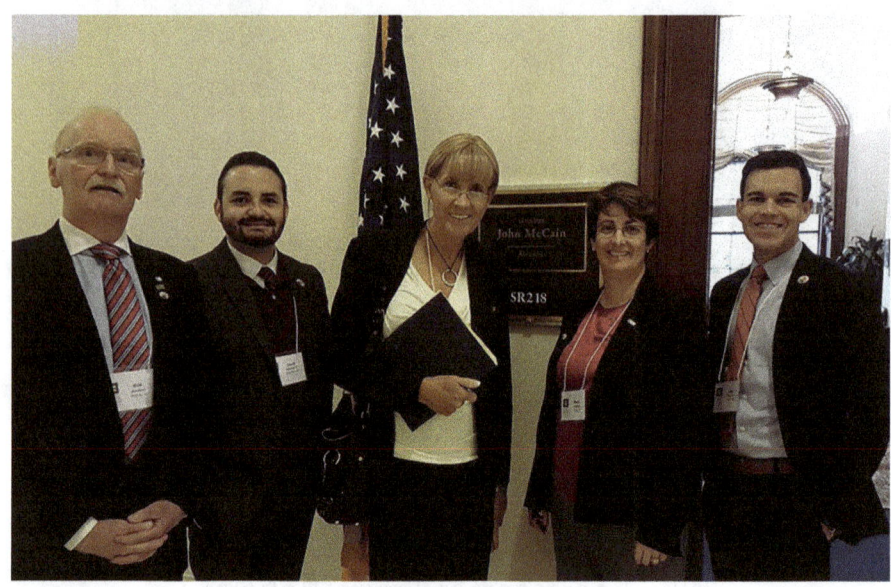

Lobbying on Capitol Hill

I had unexpectedly become a minor celebrity and used my platform to advocate for the larger transgender community.

I'm most proud of the fact that, during that entire whirlwind period, I continued to provide care for my private patients. To do this, a great deal of juggling was required. There were more than a few times when I'd make a house call, attend an interview or tee-off in a tournament, and then race home to assess yet another ill patient. This was a busy and fulfilling time.

CHAPTER TWENTY-TWO
FLYING TOO CLOSE TO THE SUN

Who is this Ann Brodie, and why does she want to take me to lunch? Apparently, she worked for the dean at McMaster Medical School; had read about my story in a magazine; liked to connect with interesting former graduates, and was attending a conference in Phoenix.

We agreed to meet for lunch at the resort where she was staying. I thought about cancelling, because I was certain that she was going to ask for a donation to the school, and Lucy and I were still struggling financially.

It was a beautiful spring day in 2017, and my life was about to take another one of those unplanned turns. Ann proved to be an engaging lunch companion, and we talked for two hours over a salad. I kept waiting for the pitch and how much the university needed financial support from alums like me—except the issue of making a donation never came up. She seemed genuinely interested in my story and wanted to learn more about transgender individuals.

As we were about to part ways, Ann announced that she wanted me to meet her husband—and that it was very important. I waited in the parking lot while she went to fetch him from their room.

It was worth the wait. Frank proved to be one of those larger-than-life individuals: an artist; irreverent; jocular; energetic, and loud. And to top it all off, he was an Irishman! And I love the Irish almost as much as I love the Italians, who were my most cherished childhood friends. The three of us made a strong connection and promised to stay in touch.

Several weeks later, Ann emailed me from Hamilton and wondered if I would be willing to talk to a friend of hers—Allyson Rowley. She was a writer and wanted to interview me for the *McMaster Alumni Magazine.*

Allyson and I spent two hours speaking on the phone, and her story—"The Butterfly Effect"—appeared in the next quarterly installment. It was masterfully written, and Ann made certain that her boss, Dean O'Byrne, had a copy on his desk. She was clearly up to something.

Dr. Paul O'Byrne read the article. Somewhere half-way through, he realized that the subject of the story—Dr. Bobbi Lancaster—had actually been Bob Lancaster, his intern back in the 1970s, during that hellish internal medicine rotation.

He wanted to meet me and asked his staff to set aside fifteen minutes the next time I visited my family in Hamilton. A month later we met, and the forty intervening years simply melted away.

We were instantly best friends again and had our picture taken together too. His eyes still crinkled shut when he smiled, like they did when he was a young man.

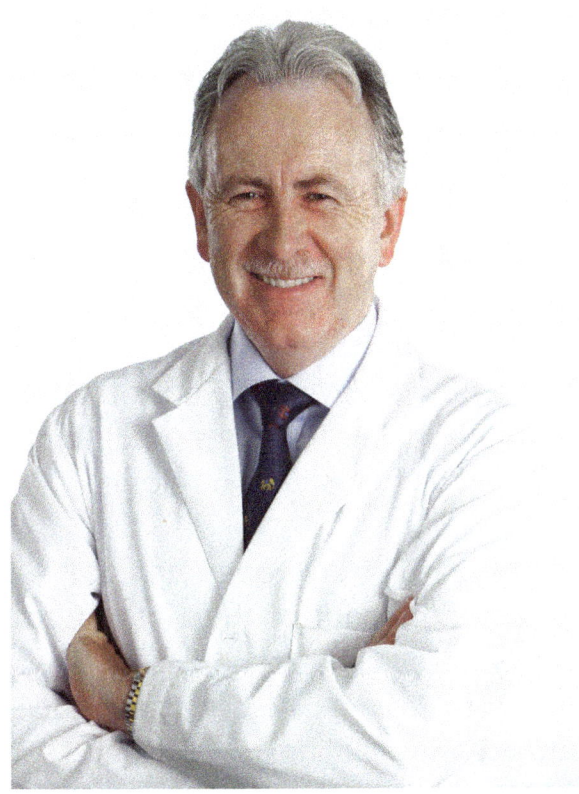

Dr. Paul O'Byrne

At the end of almost an hour, Dr. O'Byrne asked if I would consider doing a favor. The medical school had a major event for its second-year students every year—the Founders Dinner. The keynote speaker had always been one of those five individuals I introduced you to at the start of this book—the ones who'd created the program. Since Dr. Bill Walsh had recently passed away, there were no Founders left.

And so it had been decided that in the future, a graduate would be asked to speak at this prestigious event, and Dr. O'Byrne had selected me. I was initially taken aback—why me? However, I humbly accepted and couldn't wait to call Lucy, who was home in Arizona.

After the meeting, I floated over to the Faculty Club to meet with none other than Ann Brodie and Allyson Rowley. We were ecstatic that I had been chosen to deliver the keynote. I think this is what Ann had up her sleeve all along.

Later that year, on October 25, 2017—to be exact—I stood in front of the Class of 2019 and began my address. The school had flown Lucy and me in from Phoenix. Also in attendance were: my mother, my siblings and their spouses; Dean O'Byrne and his wife, Irene; many faculty members and staff; and the spouse and family of Dr. Ron McAuley—remember him? He was my mentor, and though he had died years before, I still wanted to honor all he had done for me.

My keynote was filmed and is available on Google or through the medical school website. My remarks were extremely well-received, and I was given a long standing ovation.

Transgender alumna speaks to med students

Almost 40 years ago, Robert Lancaster was an intern for chief resident Paul O'Byrne, now dean and vice-president of the Faculty of Health Sciences at McMaster University.

This fall, Bobbi Lancaster, a McMaster medical graduate of 1978, family physician in Arizona, professional golfer, author and transgender woman was the keynote speaker at the annual Founders' Dinner for the second-year students of the Michael G. DeGroote School of Medicine.

Her talk about her life, the challenges, her stumbles through medical school including guidance from the late faculty member Ronald McAuley, her career success, family and her transition at age 60 was warmly received.

"Bobbi is very courageous, a change maker who has a story that is inspirational and builds understanding. I'm very proud of her, and glad she brought her message to our students," said O'Byrne.

Her inspiring presentation is available on the Faculty of Health Sciences' YouTube channel at http://bit.ly/2AHvCWy.

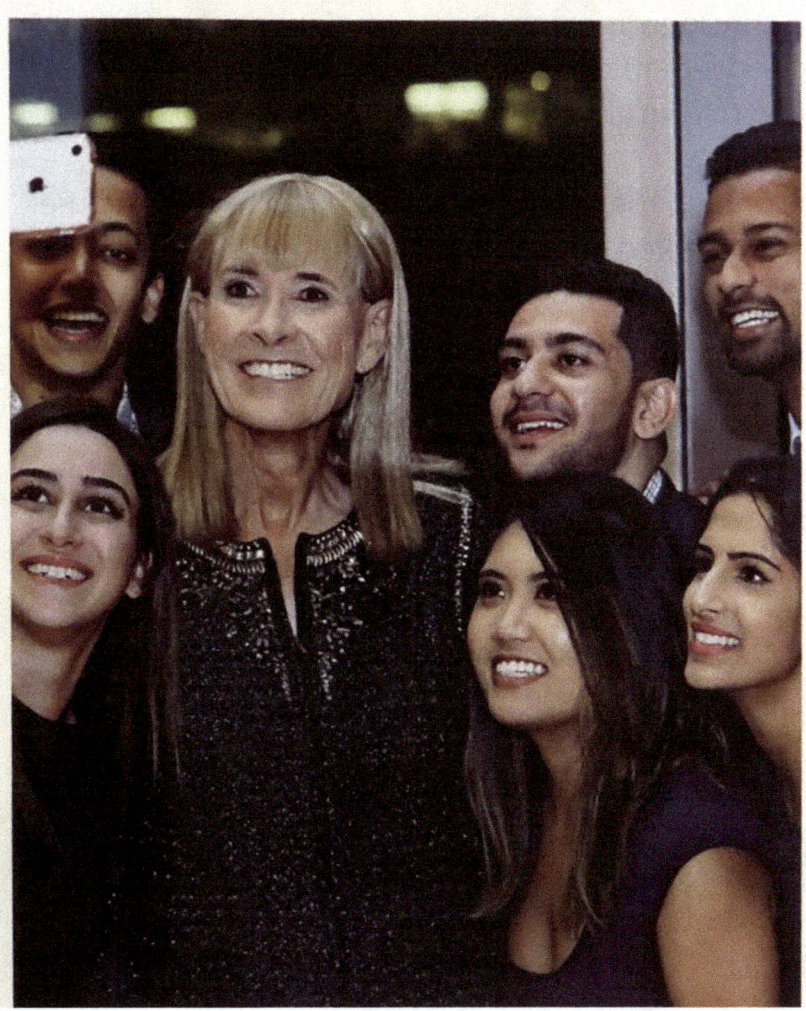

Until that moment, I didn't realize how much I had missed being around students. I had a natural gift for connecting with them; my explanations and stories about real patients were illustrative and inspirational, and my supportive nature had always been welcoming.

During the festivities, I mentioned to Dr. O'Byrne that I would give anything to be in front of a class again. I said that I could lead a tutorial group; perhaps supervise clerks and residents, or serve as a mentor. He asked if I would seriously consider moving back to Canada to teach. I replied affirmatively, and he connected me with administration and several professors.

One of the point persons was as excited as me. She talked about an associate professor position for me, which might have to be funded from several sources—the Department of Family Medicine and the School of Nursing. She noted, "We will have to be creative. However, don't worry because, based on Dr. O'Byrne's rave reviews of you, we are going to make this work."

Thus, I was tasked with reinstating my old Ontario license and Canadian Board Certification. I worked tirelessly for three months—there were multiple interactions with the College of Physicians and Surgeons of Ontario; an equal number of interactions with the Canadian College of Family Physicians; transcripts needed;

FBI and RCMP background checks; faculty and hospital privilege applications; immunizations; documentation, and even a fitting for a N95 mask in case of a pandemic.

After getting all my paperwork in order, I flew to Hamilton in late January to attend pre-arranged meetings with professors from the Department of Family Medicine. They had organized sessions with two groups of professors; a behind-the-scene tour of a teaching facility; lunch at a fancy restaurant, and finally a meeting with the department Chair.

They had no idea what this opportunity meant to me. I'd been through so much! I'd lost my jobs due to discrimination; our financial obligations had fallen on Lucy's shoulders, and this was my moment to resurrect my career and do something memorable. I could teach, and I could organize a transgender care program with the full support of the department.

The Chairman was running a little late, and he got right down to business. There was no associate professor position being created for me—there was no funding—it was a non-starter.

I could not believe what I was hearing. What in the hell was I doing here? How had I so badly misinterpreted their intent? I'd spent many months and several thousand dollars that Lucy and I could ill afford on an illusion. My mind spun as I attempted to maintain my composure. I just wanted to go home.

He continued. The Department would still like to see me involved in the program, in some capacity. I appreciated his candor and listened intently. The only path forward for me would be as an assistant clinical professor. I would receive no salary. But if I purchased a practice, I would enjoy an income stream. The Department—in time—could rotate students through my office, once I secured my patient base.

This was nuts. I was in my late sixties. I did not want to own a practice again and be responsible for a lease, staff salaries, and a thousand other things that accompany practice ownership. Not only that, I'd been gone for more than twenty-five years; the practice of medicine in Canada had changed dramatically; I only had marginal computer skills in an age when everything was done electronically; lab values were metric and completely foreign to me; there was a completely different drug formulary; all my old specialist contacts were gone, and most importantly—I would be apart from Lucy for at least a year, while she obtained her immigration papers.

Of course, I still foolishly purchased a practice. I was desperate to be a real family doctor again, and relieve Lucy of her job as the main breadwinner. I felt like I had seven more productive years left, and no one could fire me. I wanted to end my career on a high note.

Sometimes you can pursue a dream too much. There are times when a person like me can fly too close to the sun.

After an enormous amount of preparatory energy was expended, I opened the door to my first patients. Given my non-existent computer skills, it took me one hour to complete a visit that would have taken ten minutes in the paper age. I was so preoccupied typing that I could not look up and engage with the patient.

But engagement had always been my biggest strength: eye contact; observation; a touch; rapport building. And now, when I did happen to look up from the keyboard, the patient appeared guarded, questioning, and apprehensive. I had become familiar with that expression. He was trying to figure me out—male or female—he wasn't sure?

I needed Lucy, and she was 2200 miles away. I started crying and could not stop. The return of my suicidal ideation was as sudden as it was unexpected. Every cell in my body was screaming that this situation was not a good fit.

There was no time to waste. I had to return to

Arizona immediately. After hurriedly packing, I headed west toward Windsor and never looked back. Along the way, I listened to the radio and learned of the suicides of Anthony Bourdain and Kate Spade. This shocking news only made me more determined to resist the temptation and make it back home to the desert.

Several lawyers were going to be very busy cleaning up the mess I had just made—not to mention the expense and liability.

All I had wanted to do was teach. Had anybody been listening? I had a rare talent for connecting with students. I could have impacted their lives in an unbelievable way.

I just wanted to teach.

CHAPTER TWENTY-THREE
FINDING PEACE

My Gold Canyon patients were sad to learn that the teaching position had fallen through, because they knew how excited I had been. However, they were ecstatic I was back—several of them had become extremely ill.

I sensed the need for a place where I could be quiet and think. One day, I drove to a nearby state park called Boyce Thompson Arboretum. It was located thirty minutes away, next to an extinct volcano, and there was something healing about its ambience. I was drawn to the place—again and again. There were specialty tours too, where I learned about geology, Native American history, plants, bugs, bats, reptiles, birds, butterflies, and everything else to do with life.

I became hooked and wrote a book about the Arboretum called *Putting Down Roots*. Not only that, I became a volunteer—a general tour guide—and for the past seventeen months, I have mesmerized an ever-growing weekly audience with my evocative stories and facts. I also serve on the Arboretum's board of directors.

When I'm in front of twenty or thirty patrons for two hours, I connect them with nature in a powerful way. Perhaps one of them will be inspired to oppose the forces that are working against the health of our planet.

Sometimes I close my eyes and pretend that I'm addressing a group of medical students—bringing clarity to their patient management decisions, and demonstrating best practice around empathy and communication techniques.

A person can always dream.

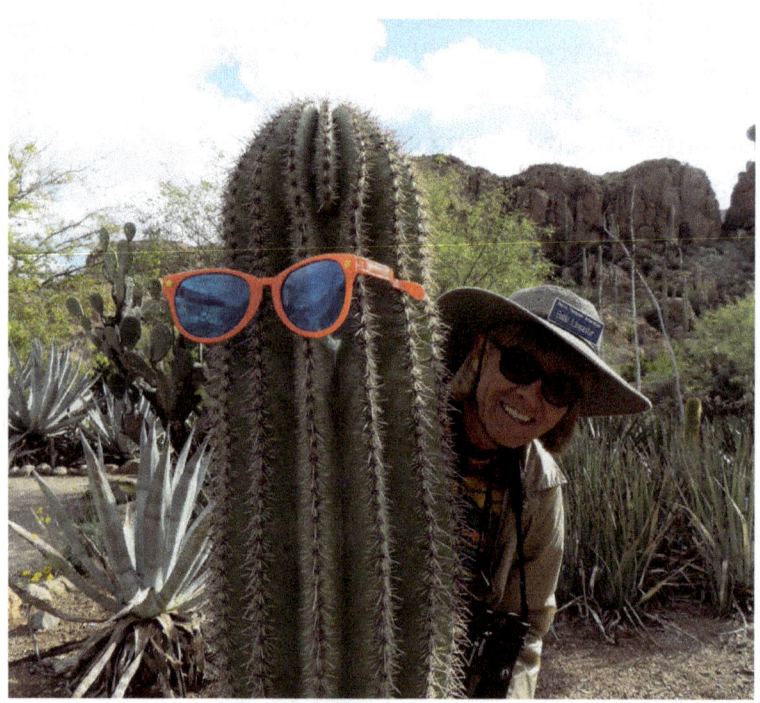

Bobbi, the tour guide,
with her special friend—Gus.

CHAPTER TWENTY-FOUR
TIME TO SAY GOODBYE

We've made it to the final chapter together, and I can only guess who my companions have been. I know Dr. O'Byrne is one of them. After all, he agreed to write the foreword. Perhaps some are old classmates, who wanted to reminisce about the way we were. Maybe there are some curious medical students, eager to learn more about the path they have embarked upon. Possibly, there are young people contemplating a medical career.

My hunch is there are also a number of my old patients who are thrilled to have reconnected with me—by way of this book—and want to see if I mentioned them in any of my stories. Others may be academics, administrators, or historians—eager to make certain I had my facts correct and did not misrepresent the program in any way.

The telling of some of my more interesting patient encounters has been an honor. Recounting events around my tutorials, clerkship, and residency has run the gamut of the human experience: triumph; defeat; elation; profound sadness; insignificance; life-altering.

The revolutionary new approach to medical

education—created fifty years ago at McMaster by the Founding Fathers—continues to be deservedly applauded. And its impact cannot be overstated.

One can only guess at the next new breakthrough. Is there a young version of Dr. John Evans in our midst right now, dreaming of yet another new approach to education and the delivery of medical care? My guess is that it will involve artificial intelligence.

However, no matter what the new paradigm, helping people will always be a profoundly human experience. It will continue to involve empathetic caregivers. And in my opinion, there needs to be more effort to ensure that the provider remains healthy too. The adverse outcomes I've observed in myself and in many of my colleagues are unacceptable.

My classmates and I received the most brilliant instructions around self-direction and critical thinking. And yet, we received no training in crucial areas such as: self-care; work-life balance; burnout; team dynamics; information on our own personal strengths and weaknesses; how to operate a practice; money management, and the choice of a specialty. The list is long.

Perhaps the McMaster curriculum is now addressing these issues. If not, I hope there is a visionary—some new change-maker—who will build upon McMaster's incredible strengths, and create a more humane caregiver training approach. This will produce graduates that remain healthy and productive throughout a long career.

***

Sometimes I'm asked if there is a lesson or two I was taught during my medical school training that has stuck with me. Is there a message that really resonates and that I rely upon, even now, to confront a challenge?

The question forced me to reflect on all the education I've received—from kindergarten to the completion of my undergraduate degree. Of course there were mathematical equations; the laws of physics; chemical reactions; memorized dates in history; geographical locations of places that I'll never visit; Latin verses; Shakespearean sonnets, and so much more. But to be honest, I've forgotten most of that stuff a long time ago.

On the other hand, the most impactful lessons I've learned come from McMaster. The curriculum did not just require me to memorize facts. It taught me how to teach myself, and provided me with the tools that I needed to cut through the clutter, and identify the nugget—otherwise called evidence-based truth. The program gave me permission to think outside the box. My tutorial group classmates embraced my off-the-wall suggestions.

I'll leave you with two stories that illustrate what I'm talking about.

The first concerns an incident that occurred a few months ago. Lucy and I had returned home from a busy day at our respective jobs. We entered the kitchen and were greeted by the sound of frantic scratching. It was emanating from the hood above our stove. An animal had become trapped inside—it had likely entered the vent on the roof and tumbled down into the appliance.

The animal had to be rescued. It was a perfect problem-based conundrum, designed for my medical school tutorial group many years ago. Neither one of us possessed the skills to dismantle the hood, so I called our builder—Ken. It was a Friday evening, and he had left for California. Ken would be back Monday morning to remove the appliance and rescue the trapped occupant—if it were still alive. Lucy and I tried to imagine another plan, and we were definitely thinking outside the box.

We listened to the on-and-off scratching all day Saturday, and by Sunday it was weaker and less frequent. I couldn't stand it anymore. I told Lucy about a solution that had appeared from somewhere in my brain. I was going to tie a bolt to the end of a long piece of twine, climb onto the roof, locate the vent, and lower the string to the hood below. The animal would realize it was being rescued, cling to this life preserver and be pulled to safety.

My tutorial group would have applauded the idea. Lucy was more skeptical. However, there was nothing to lose.

I climbed up to the roof while clutching the string with the bolt attached. I lowered this last resort contraption down the vent, sat on a parapet, and waited for something… anything.

Nothing happened, and my mind wandered to another place and time. I was reminded of the many days that I went fishing with my father as a child. It was just the two of us, sitting quietly in the boat, being rocked to sleep by the gentle waves… waiting for a nibble. If I strained, I could still hear the silence.

And then the spell was broken by a movement— a nibble—barely noticeable at first, and then more insistent.

I slowly pulled the twine from the depths of the kitchen below. The string felt heavier, and my heart raced from anticipation.

And then it appeared—a cactus wren—gripping the bolt with both feet, as if its life were in the balance. The bird stepped from the bolt onto the little structure above the vent and perched. It was dehydrated and completely exhausted.

We looked at each other, and neither one of us could break from the connection we made. I began to cry. I had saved a life, and that does not happen every day—even for a family doctor.

At least three minutes passed. I wondered if the bird might actually be on the verge of death, given the ordeal it had been through.

And then another wren landed nearby—its mate—and nudged its rescued partner. That's all it took. There was a blur of flapping wings and then they were off, hopefully to a happier future.

My imagined tutorial group applauded in the background.

***

My final story revolves around a recent incident that took place on a quiet Arizona morning.

Our neighbors were vacationing, and they had asked me to look after their terrier—Ruffian. It was pre-dawn as we strolled down the shoulder of the road.

The Doctor Is In

Ruffian tugged at the leash—he had to pee—and we diverted to a nearby bush. He lifted his leg and was going about his business when I looked down. I noticed the dog was urinating on a desert cottontail rabbit that had chosen that very place as its overnight shelter.

The rabbit looked directly at me and silently pleaded that I not divulge its location. The dog lowered its leg, spotted the rabbit, and lunged.

But the cottontail was too quick. It swiftly raced down the street and dodged—directly into the path of an oncoming car.

I could hear the thump, followed by a thump again. The rabbit's body was crushed. However, it was still conscious and looked at me with those same beautiful dark eyes. I lingered briefly and then turned away—there was nothing more I could do.

And then Shirley Hurst and Vince Rudnick both appeared from somewhere deep inside. They reminded me that when it seems like there is nothing more to do, that's the moment you are especially needed. It's when you'll provide your most exquisite care.

I turned and walked back to the scene of the accident. The rabbit was still conscious, and those eyes betrayed its fear. Another car was approaching, and the rabbit could not get away. Was it going to be struck again, or would it be run over by the next car—or the next one after that?

I would have been distressed too.

Bending down, I picked up the damaged little body and placed it under a nearby tree. Death was inevitable, yes, but at least it would not be terrified of ongoing injury during its last few minutes of life.

Ruffian and I stood watch, like a pair of unlikely bodyguards. There we were—three passengers on this spaceship called earth—and one of us was about to give up a seat.

The rabbit took its final breath.

In my mind's eye, I spotted Shirley and Vince to the left of the tree, nodding their heads in approval. It had been such a simple thing to do, but I had provided much needed palliative care for that little creature during its final moments.

I looked at the tree again, and they were gone—until the next time.

***

I hope these last two stories have illustrated the powerful impact that the McMaster Medical

School training has had on my life. The lessons have been internalized, and sometimes it's hard to know where McMaster ends and where Bobbi begins.

And now it's time for a final handshake and a hug. It's hard to say goodbye because we've been through so much together. However, I've run out of words, and to be honest, I think I've shared enough. Besides, I have a patient in need of a house call—this doctor is in today.

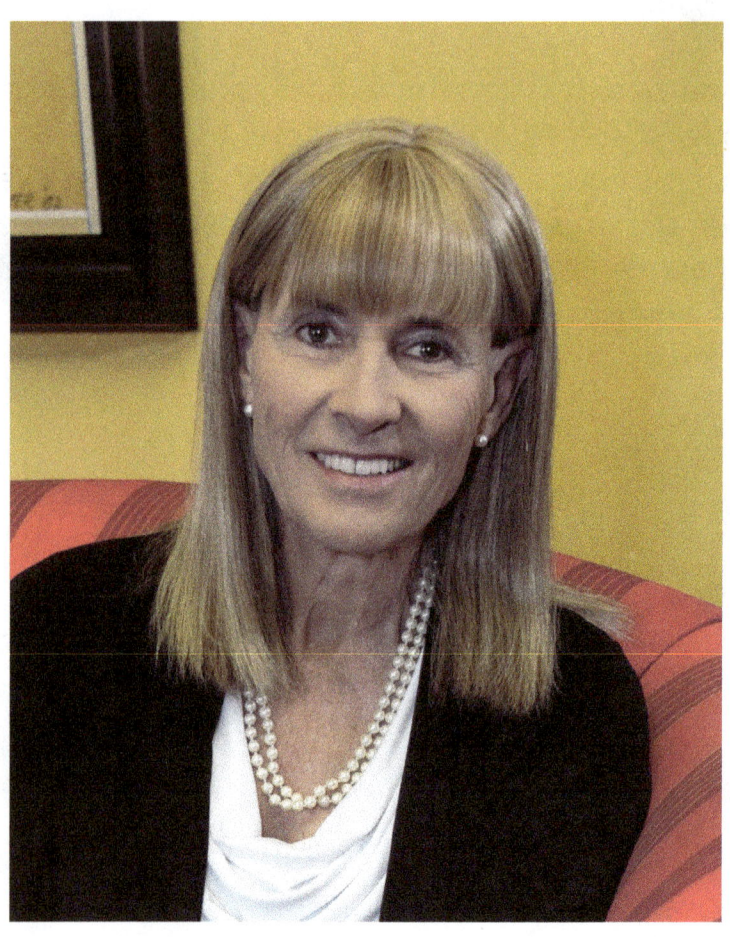

ABOUT THE AUTHOR

Dr. Bobbi Lancaster is a family physician and a proud graduate of McMaster University Medical School in 1978.

Bobbi resides in Gold Canyon, Arizona, and enjoys a rich and rewarding life with her wife, Lucy. She is an author, speaker, and transgender rights advocate. Bobbi also volunteers a great deal of time at Boyce Thompson Arboretum where she leads general tours and serves on its board of directors. The garden is a ninety-five year old, nationally acclaimed treasure—smack in the middle of the Sonoran desert. It features an extinct volcano; lava flows throughout; a canyon and riparian area, and dry land plants from all over the world.

She is also a retired professional golfer and, at one time, an accomplished pianist. Bobbi only occasionally plays golf now and hasn't sat at a keyboard in years. There are simply too many other things to do.

Aside from staying fit and hiking in the surrounding desert landscape, Bobbi serves as the Principal Poop Scooper around the house. She was given this title by Lucy, who—when she's not seeing patients as a nurse practitioner—is a renowned Havanese dog breeder. Bobbi enjoys the work, and says that it keeps her grounded.

The Doctor Is In

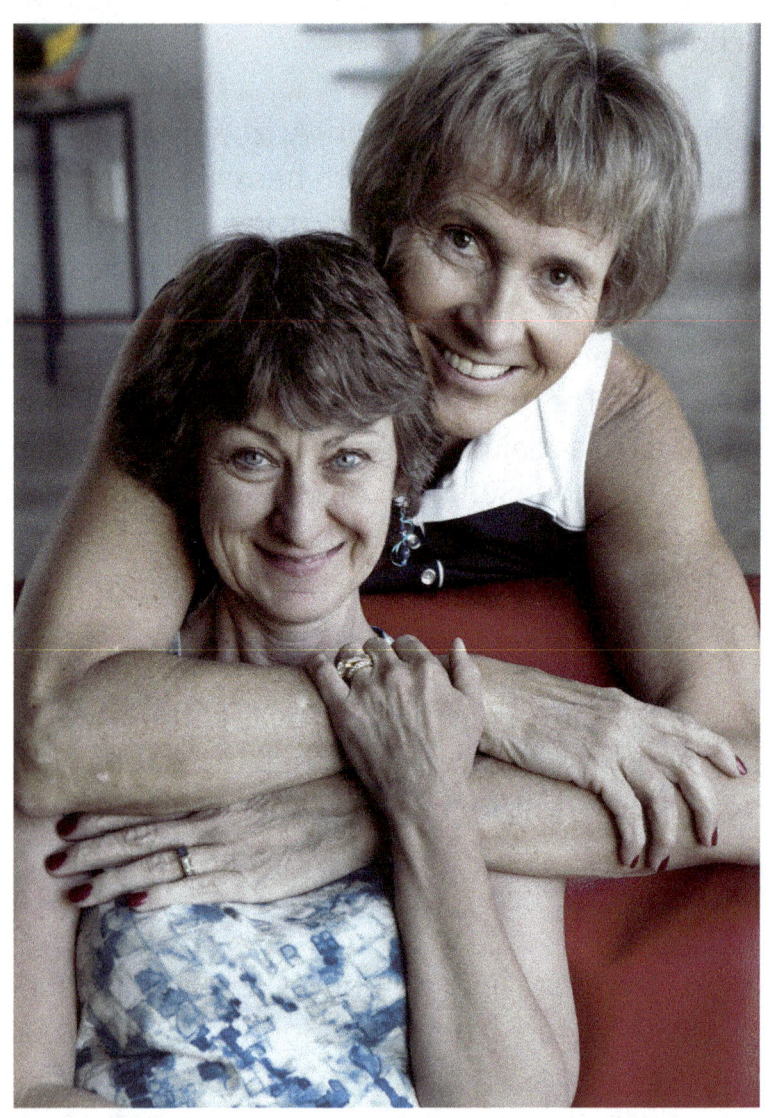

The Doctor Is In

After thoroughly washing her hands of course, Bobbi continues to provide care for a group of patients in the area. This work keeps her fulfilled.

Dr. Lancaster can be reached at:
plusoneatsixty@hotmail.com.

The Doctor Is In

ACKNOWLEDGEMENTS

There are countless people to thank, all of whom contributed to my career and the writing of this book. I won't attempt to mention every patient, professor, friend, and family member responsible. Inevitably, someone would be unintentionally left off the list—feelings could be hurt. Nevertheless, when all is said and done, I have been deeply influenced by their collective teaching and love. They have cared about me as much as I have cared for them. However, there are several individuals I must acknowledge.

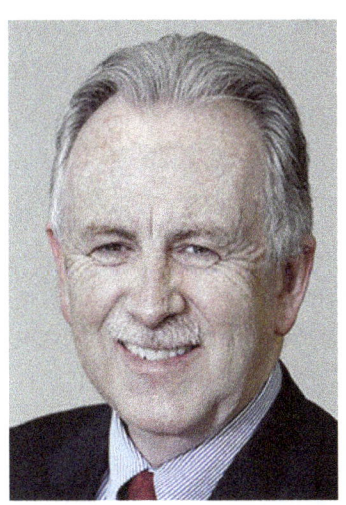

Dr. Paul O'Byrne
The current Dean and Vice President of the Michael G. DeGroote School of Medicine—formerly called McMaster Medical School. He is a world-renowned expert in the field of pulmonology.

Dr. O'Byrne has published more than 400 peer-reviewed studies, authored 100 review papers and edited ten books. These are mind-boggling numbers! Even more remarkable, he remains the same humble, self-effacing, and readily approachable person I met forty years ago.

Dr. O'Byrne, for some unfathomable reason, asked me to be the first non-Founder to address the second year medical students at their annual dinner in 2017. He did this even though he had never heard me deliver a speech, and he had thousands of alums to choose from. As it turned out, my address was hugely applauded. But, how did he know my speech would be relevant and that I would not stumble and be overwhelmed by the moment?

And then several months ago, I called to ask if he would review this book. Not only that, I asked if he would provide a foreword once he read it. Dr. O'Byrne agreed to write an introduction even before glancing at the manuscript! I appreciate his confidence in me, more than I can say.

Dr. O'Byrne reminds me of Dr. Ron McAuley. Their combined support has propelled me to achieve goals that I thought were unattainable. Paul, as he likes to be called, is one of the most extraordinary persons I have ever met. Perhaps everyone who meets him says exactly the same thing. It wouldn't surprise me.

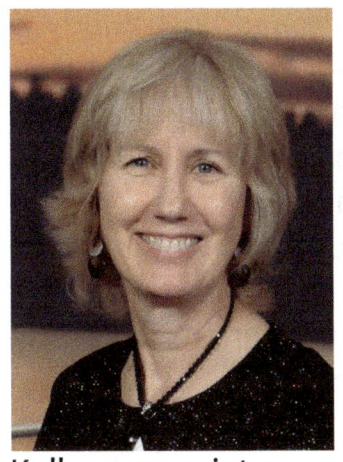

Kally Reynolds
An accomplished writer, author, editor, educator, life coach, and a public relations professional. She lives in my community and has edited several of my recent books.

Kally appreciates my vulnerable story-telling, messaging, and voice. She happily performed the tedious work of editing this manuscript because she strongly believes *The Doctor Is In* will be both helpful and entertaining for all readers. Kally can be reached at: *coachkally@gmail.com*.

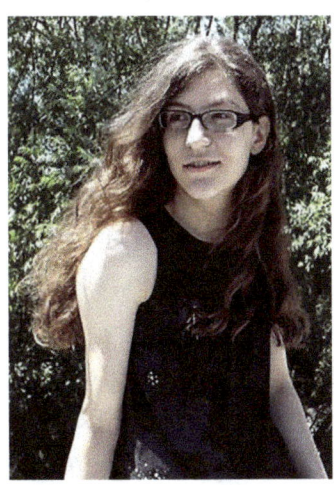

Jackie Casey
Impressively creative and devoted to supporting my writing. She designed the cover and formatted the book for publication. She also resides in the Gold Canyon community.

Jackie has a fine arts degree in comic art, and her enthusiasm and positive energy are contagious. Jackie can be reached at *jecruby@gmail.com*.

I must acknowledge my wife and best buddy—Lucy. She is the recipient of my constant grammatical uncertainty and questions about spelling. In fact, I have bombarded her with frequent requests to spell check, Photoshop, and scan documents. Lucy is delighted when I leave to see patients, play golf, or lead a tour at the Arboretum. It allows her to luxuriate for a few hours of well-deserved silence.

In addition, the residents of Westdale, who had their homes expropriated for the purpose of building the medical school, deserve honorable mention too. I assume that they were fairly compensated for the disruption this initiative caused. It was for the greater good, and people around the world have been helped because of their sacrifice.

I would be remiss in not thanking Clare Crozier, the surviving husband of Shirley Hurst. He very graciously provided me with many photos and background information about this remarkable woman.

Joan McAuley and her children also furnished me with memorable anecdotes and treasured pictures of Ron—he passed away many years ago. They attended several large assemblies where I was the guest speaker, and it afforded me the opportunity to express my gratitude for Dr. McAuley through them.

Finally, McMaster Medical School was built on land once occupied by indigenous people. I have become painfully aware of the disruption that the Euro-Canadian intruders created when they claimed the landscape as their own many years ago. My classmates and I had unknowingly met on the traditional territories of the Mississauga and Haudenosaunee nations, and on the lands protected by the "Dish With One Spoon" wampum agreement. Respectfully, I hope their descendants will read this book, appreciate our gratitude, and perhaps conclude that great good came from their ancestral suffering.

CPSIA information can be obtained
at www.ICGtesting.com
Printed in the USA
LVHW061411150920
665921LV00005B/1